HERBS
& OTHER MEDICINAL PLANTS

With an introduction by Jerry Cowhig

**ORBIS BOOKS
LONDON**

Contents

3   Foreword
5   Herbalism and medicine
5   The language of herbs
6   Spices and drugs
6   Collection and drying
8   Drug preservation
9   Active principles
10 Types of medicine
11 How much to take?
11 Medicinal foods
12 Wild and exotic plants
13 Not just for drugs
14 Summary
14 Bibliography
15 Glossary of terms
17 Illustrations

All illustrations were photographed by Mirella Bavestrelli, with the exception of plate 66 (by ARDEA Photographics) and plate 81 (by Aldus Books)

Based on the Italian of Carlo d'Andreta

© Istituto Geografico De Agostini, Novara 1968
Introduction © Orbis Publishing Limited, London 1972
Printed in Italy by IGDA, Novara
SBN 0 85613 116 4

This is a book about the power of plants, and how that power can be harvested and utilized. It is for everyone who has never thought of plants as useful except by virtue of their beauty and their value in the obvious, 'large-scale' ways: for instance as timber, food or fibre. And it is also for that increasing group of people who are turning to the old, 'natural' means of health, through herbal foods and medicines, and for whom an illustrated guide to the important medicinal species may be of real interest and practical use.

In the Western world today there are numerous pharmaceutical companies, many of them with an annual research budget in the millions of dollars, not to mention their sales turnover, who can provide sterile injections, pills, lotions, drips and ointments for nearly every condition that their medical colleagues can diagnose. In this vastly streamlined technology, what place is there for the herbal remedy?

A close look at this question reveals the simple solution that there is, in fact, no basis for competition between modern and herbal therapeutics; we are talking about one and the same line of work – the use of Nature's best resources to combat disease. For the drug industry itself, sophisticated though it may be, relies very heavily on plants for its medicinal preparations. Many of the plants described in this book are cultivated on a large scale by the industry, which needs them for their active constituents. In other cases, where chemists are able to make drugs in the laboratory, the drugs they make are often based on natural substances; simple herbal cures are adopted and adapted, as more is learned about the chemistry of natural compounds and the pharmacological action of such compounds in the human body.

Nevertheless, there are people who align themselves on the two ends of a pharmacognostic tug-of-war rope: some saying that herbal medicines are the only true and heaven-sent means to a full natural health; and their opponents maintaining that such a view is cranky nonsense and that the use of herbals is antiquated, ineffective quackery. Only the synthetic medicines of today, they say, can be of any use in therapeutics. The truth, of course, lies with neither of these extreme views, and the aim of this book is to describe some plants which are and have been used with benefit, and in what ways.

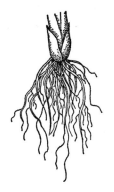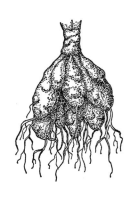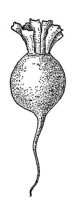

Three types of true root: fibrous, tuberous, and tap-root.

Herbalism and medicine

Herbalism is a subject with a long history. We know that animals in various kinds of trouble can turn to plants which they know will cure them, and it is probable that primitive man happened on cures in much the same way: by trial and error, the results being passed on from one generation to the next; and, perhaps, to some extent by instinct. Certainly, the same archeological evidence that tells us of early man's exploitation of plants for food, fuel, tools and building materials, also shows us that he had a battery of herbal cures for his common ailments. Of course there were mythical sidetracks, for example the idea that the shape of a plant indicated its curative value. This, the doctrine of signatures, supposed that a plant with liver-shaped leaves (*Anemone hepatica*) would cure liver disease, and that *Physalis alkakengi* was equally predestined to alleviate complaints of the bladder because of the balloon shape of the calyx around its fruit. Such a doctrine was inevitably discredited, to the extent that herbalism fell into disrepute.

But it is from the ancient herbals that our modern pharmacopeias have developed, just as modern chemistry owes its foundations to alchemy, and medicine to many strange and misplaced practices! Moreover, the herbal is not so outdated as those analogies may make it sound. The number of people, in all countries of the world, who rely wholly or partly on herbal cures, and the measure of success they achieve, illustrates its modern position.

At this time, however, a word of warning is essential. The plants described in this book are valuable only because they contain powerful chemical ingredients, and for that same reason they can be dangerous. Prepared and used properly, by a pharmacist or a trained herbalist, they can provide medicines that are unlikely to be hazardous; but in the majority of cases they are not suitable for home medication. Mistakes can occur, and may be tragic. Remember that when our grandmothers use herbal mixtures, they are working on a lifetime's experience; the herbalist, too, has his training, more

intensive and detailed. Everyone can benefit from the role that medicinal plants play today, but not usually by setting up his own practice!

This warning applies particularly to parents of young children. Few would risk a herbal experiment on the family, but the wise parent also protects the child from his own innocence, keeping him away from dangerous plants.

The language of herbs

This book is not for the specialist, but for the layman with no more than a smattering of knowledge in either botany or medicine. As far as botany is concerned, it is necessary only to know the various parts of a plant (berry, rhizome, etc), which are explained in the introductory text, and to understand how plants are named and identified. Obviously the simplest way to name plants is by common names, like 'hogweed' or 'red clover', but unfortunately the exclusive use of these casual names can lead to a great deal of confusion, because they vary from country to country, and even in different areas of any single country. Therefore, although common names are used in this book, the recognized Latin names are given in addition. These are always double-barrelled names: the first identifying the genus; the second, the species. For example, the various types of foxglove all fall within one genus, of which the generic name is *Digitalis*. Each species of foxglove then has its own specific name, such as *Digitalis purpurea* or *D. lutea.* Such generic and specific names are always printed in italics, and the genus may be abbreviated to a single capital letter when the meaning is obvious, as in the example above.

The use of medical terms can be justified in much the same way: they may seem intimidating, but have the advantages of conciseness and accuracy. In fact, there are not many unfamiliar medical terms in this book, partly because the history and development of herbal medicines has been concerned with conditions and cures that are familiar to everyone. In other words, it is concerned with things like fever and constipation, and less with the

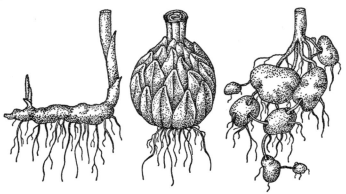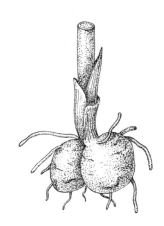

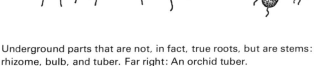

Underground parts that are not, in fact, true roots, but are stems:
rhizome, bulb, and tuber. Far right: An orchid tuber.

newly discovered diseases with long names. Nevertheless,
a glossary is printed at the end of this introductory text,
to define the technical terms that are used in the book,
both medical and botanical.

Spices and drugs

There is no strict dividing line that separates the various
plant products. We name them according to the use we
make of them, in our society or in our bodies. Starch may
be a food or an addition to our laundry: to the plant, it is
still starch.

So it is with drugs and spices. The latter are those
extracts of plants that we choose to employ as flavours,
for example nutmeg, pepper and cinnamon, but they
could equally well be called medicines, as all three of the
examples given have some pharmacological action. The
same applies to many of the plants illustrated in this book,
while in other cases the plants are used solely for
medicinal purposes, either because they are not desirable
kitchen ingredients or because they are dangerous.

In order to be called a drug, a substance must have the
property of alleviating disease. It may actually cure the
disease, although this is only true of such once-for-all
agents as the antibiotics. More often it helps the body to
fight the disease in some way or, as in the case of most
herbal medicines, benefits the patient by relieving the
symptoms. Also the word 'drug' should be restricted to
substances that have been prepared in some way and are
dispensed in a standardized form and potency. Thus, it
cannot invariably be applied to the results of crude
extraction procedures, which are better called 'crude
drugs'. In any mixture, the component with the
pharmacological effect is called the 'active principle',
although in herbal mixtures there may be several of
these, with varying degrees of importance.

Plants which provide crude drugs are often recognized
as such in the specific name *officinalis*, which indicates that
they have at some time had official recognition. All plants
that have some medicinal properties (whether or not they
have the historical tag of *officinalis*) are listed in a
pharmacopeia, along with all the other medicines in use.
Every country has its own pharmacopeia, or makes use of
the International Pharmacopeia, and it may come as a
surprise to the opponents of herbal medicine to see how
many medicinal plants feature in these works. However,
the pharmacopeias of different countries do not always
contain the same plants; broadly speaking they do, but
there are many plants that are recognized in one country
but not in another, either because of local availability or,
more probably today, because of different interpretations
of their importance by the compilers of the
pharmacopeias. Naturally, these reference works are
revised regularly, and the official status of medicinal
plants is subject to change.

It is worth mentioning that, to a botanist, the term
'herb' means a plant that has no woody stem above the
ground, while a herbalist uses the word to mean only
those parts of such a plant that are actually visible above
ground, or the leafy tips of other, woody plants. In general
usage, however, the word herb describes any plant that is
used medicinally (or, indeed, in cookery, though these
usually are 'true herbs'). In this book, the word is used in
this loosest sense, and 'herbal' is taken to mean any crude
extract of a plant which has medicinal properties.

Collection and drying

The collection of medicinal plants is a matter of
considerable care and skill, for several reasons. Above all,
of course, it is essential to collect the right species of
plant, which requires a knowledge of botanical
identification. The illustrations in ancient herbals were
made for this reason, enabling people to identify plants
simply and surely, even when there was no adequate
written description; for the consequences of an error in
collection can be tragic.

The question of identity does not arise so often today,
however, because few people (quite rightly) attempt to
pick flowers for their own medicinal uses. On some

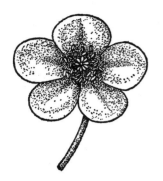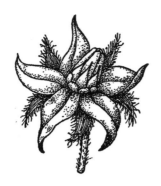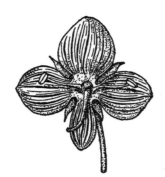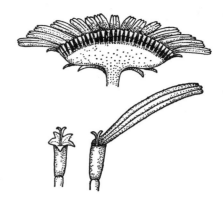

The grouping of petals is called the corolla, and may be in many forms: the buttercup has separate petals; borage is gamopetalous.

Veronica is also gamopetalous (petals united); finally, the compound head of the daisy has two types of petal – ray and disc.

occasions when this is done, mistakes are still made. Most commercial supplies of medicinal plants are, in fact, cultivated under standard conditions in the USA, Europe and the Far East. Some are available for home extraction, while others are legally controlled as regards sale and possession. Another legal point, apart from the protection of the public, is that in some areas plants have been picked for their medicinal properties to such an extent that they have become scarce, and the law has stepped in to conserve them. Examples of this are the edelweiss and gentian, in parts of Europe.

Just as with food plants, the time of harvesting medicinal plants is of considerable importance. Simply knowing which part of the plant holds the active principle is not enough; the amount of it in the plant will vary with the seasons – just like edible fruits, which become sweeter, then begin to deteriorate – and the herbalist's purpose is most efficiently served by collection of the plant at a time when it is at its most potent. Quite commonly, this is the time when the part to be collected is at full maturity.

The experienced grower of herbal plants also observes other practices, in order to achieve the most reliable effect from his products. For example, it is best to gather the plants in warm, dry weather, when there is no dew. Moreover, different parts of plants require different methods of collection and drying, and must be considered separately.

Beginning with the parts that grow underground, it must be remembered that these are not all roots, although they are often referred to as such, in popular usage. In fact, many are modified stems, including tubers (for example, the potato), rhizomes (rhubarb), and bulbs (onion). Whatever type of underground growth is to be collected, the plant must be pulled out of the ground with care, causing as little damage as possible. The roots, or other parts, must then be cleaned of the soil that adheres to them. Sandy soil may be shaken off, but when the soil contains clay, the plant must be washed carefully and dried at once.

Large roots are sometimes cut into smaller pieces, and

the next step is to place all the clean parts on a cloth to dry. Traditionally, drying was done in the sun, but today ovens are set to controlled temperatures, usually in the region of 50°C, and the roots or rhizomes put there to dry. The drying is a critical step in the preparation of herbs, because the presence of any residual moisture will encourage the growth of moulds, leading in turn to the deterioration of the plant and the destruction of its active principles.

Collection of roots and other underground parts of annual plants is usually done just before the plant is due to flower, while for others the best time is autumn and winter. There are always exceptions to this kind of rule-of-thumb: for example, the tubers of orchids and the rhizomes of the male fern are collected in summer.

Turning to the aerial, or overground, parts of a plant, the bark is removed from branches that are at least two years old, and is usually taken in either autumn or spring. In autumn, it can be cut easily from the branch, using a knife. In spring, however, it is more successful to make two circular cuts, a few inches apart, and a third one along the bark to release it. This technique releases a complete ring of bark, which is then dried in the same manner as underground parts.

Buds, not surprisingly, have to be gathered at springtime, when they have started to develop but have not yet opened. They need to be dried very carefully, in the shade rather than in the open sunshine, and not in a heated oven. The same care must be applied to the drying of leaves, which are usually collected in the growing season (although there are exceptions: mallow leaves, for instance, are collected when the plant is in flower). Leaves have to be chosen carefully; any that are yellow, partially eaten or showing signs of disease must be rejected.

True herbs – by definition plants that have no woody stem above the ground – are collected at the start of the flowering season. Again, the damaged or yellow parts are thrown away, and the plant is dried in the same manner as for buds.

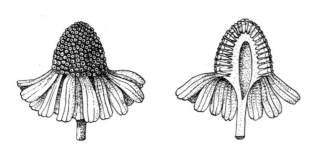

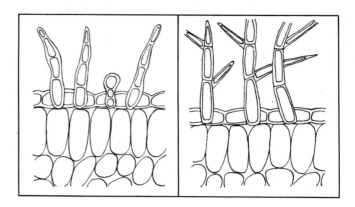

Mature head of chamomile, whole and in section. Outside are the ray florets, and inside are the disc florets, with smaller petals.

The leaves of foxglove (left) can be confused with those of the mulleins (right), but microscopic examination shows different hairs.

Most flowers are collected when they are open, although some, like the hawthorn and chamomile, can be gathered as buds and allowed to open later. In any case, the collection is usually done in the morning, after the dew has evaporated. Before drying, some parts of the flower may be rejected. Often this is the case with the peduncle, or stalk, and in other cases the sepals (calyx) are removed, when the active principle is contained in the petals (corolla). The drying of flowers requires as much care as that of buds, because of their delicacy.

Fleshy fruits are usually collected when they are fully ripe; in most cases this is the time when the chemical changes in the fruit have reached a stage where the active principles are at their highest concentration. On the other hand, strawberries, raspberries, bilberries and mulberries are more potent when gathered a short time before their fullest ripeness. Dry, dehiscent fruits are best collected when they are ripe but before they have dried out on the plant. The collection of dry, indehiscent fruits depends on whether the crude drug is obtained from the whole fruit or only from the seeds: if it is throughout the fruit, collection is carried out before it reaches maturity; otherwise, when only the seeds are a source of the active principle, they are allowed to become fully ripe.

Finally, the seeds of pulpy fruits, such as gourds, marrows and quinces, are gathered just before the fruit is fully ripe. The small seeds of dry fruits are also collected before full maturity, at the same time as the plant. Then, after drying, they are obtained merely by shaking the plant.

Drug preservation

Inevitably, there is a lapse of time between when the plant is collected and when the drug is extracted from it, and the preservation of the plant tissue during this period is of major importance. Harvested plants are not dead, but continue in their internal chemical activity. (This is equally true of the fruits and vegetables which one buys in the shops, whereas a piece of meat, on the other hand,

is quite dead.) Therefore one has to take account of the undesirable changes that can take place in medicinal plants, and to arrange their storage and preservation in such a way as to minimize these changes. Furthermore, the possibility of attack by other species – micro-organisms, insects and animals – must be guarded against.

The first, and most vital preservative technique is the drying, already described. As long as the moisture content is below 10 per cent, enzymes in the plant are virtually inactive and cannot cause undesirable changes. Also, the growth of micro-organisms, particularly moulds, needs some moisture; drying plants and storing them in conditions of low humidity protects against this possibility. Even in an apparently dry place, some plants absorb tiny amounts of moisture very readily, and special containers have to be used. These have a false base, perforated so that water vapour is absorbed by the quicklime placed below on the solid base. However, it is sufficient to store most species in polythene bags.

Light and air may also encourage the deterioration of some species; the bag keeps out fresh air, and storage in the dark rules out any chance of photochemical changes, which can discolour the plant and cause deterioration of the active principles.

Protection from attack by insects and rodents is essential for plants which are poisonous to man; often they are not harmful to these animals. The tubers of aconite, or monkshood, are an example of this difference. Insects often attack plants that contain nutritive substances, for example rhizomes or tubers containing starch, soiling them with their droppings, and hollowing out channels in the tissues. Rats, too, will work their way through almost any stored plant material, and the only protection against them is to store the plant in glass or metal containers.

With these precautions, some herbs will keep almost indefinitely; it is not unknown for active alkaloids to be extracted from samples after 300 years of storage. Some species, on the other hand, have a limited storage life, particularly when they contain volatile oils.

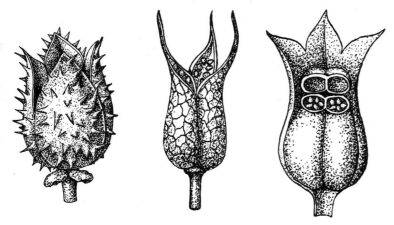

More identifying parts of individual plants: open thorn-apple fruit; follicle of the aconite (monkshood) fruit; section of henbane flower.

Active principles

Plants contain numerous different kinds of chemical compounds, in small and large amounts, varying greatly or in minute detail between one species and the next. The most fundamental chemical reaction that a plant is capable of – and also the one phenomenon on which all life on Earth depends – is the process of photosynthesis: the plant absorbs water and carbon dioxide, and uses the energy of sunlight to build carbohydrates from these simple starting materials. For this reason, all plants contain some sugar or starch, or related substances, and in some cases these are used by man, either for food or for medicinal purposes.

Sugar cane, sugar beet, root crops including the potato, and cereals are examples of such crops that man harvests for food, while other, similar, plants can be used therapeutically. Some tubers, for example, contain a substance called inulin, which is closely related to starch, and which is used in herbal preparations.

Another major nutrient produced by plants is fat – or rather, oil. Many seeds contain large quantities of oil, both in the seed coats and in the kernels, and extraction of this is very important commercially – never more so than today, now that unsaturated oils are regarded as healthier than hard animal fats. Some of these oils have medicinal uses apart from their nutritive value, and some, such as castor oil, are used mainly for medicinal purposes.

Apart from these nutritive substances, which man can use for energy or for their pharmacological effects, plants contain many types of chemical compounds with the ability to affect the human body. The bulk of herbal remedies, in fact, rely on fairly small quantities of extremely powerful substances for their pharmacological actions. The active principles are many and varied, but nevertheless it is possible to list the main chemical types.

Acids are often present in plant tissues, particularly fruits, and they have a number of important properties. In herbal medicine, their astringency is commonly harnessed, but in addition to this some properties are specific to individual acids: for example, ascorbic and citric acid in citrus fruits; oxalic acid in rhubarb.

Certain parts of plants, particularly seeds such as linseed, will produce *mucilage* when placed in hot water. This sticky, semi-transparent substance is used as an emollient. Another sticky, viscous product of plants is *gum*, which is usually the plant's response to injury or infection, and which has been found very useful to man. The food industry consumes large quantities of several different gums every year, because of their ability to act as fillers and stabilizers. Medicinally they can fulfil the same role, in making up pills and pastilles, or can act in their own right; some, for example, may be taken to alleviate diarrhea.

The reason why green figs are unpalatable is that they produce a white, acrid, milky substance; this is another type of raw drug, called a *latex*, consisting of starch, gums, resins, and other substances, suspended in water to give the white mixture. The latex produced by some plants is of pharmacological importance, such as that of opium, while others, such as rubber, have a value to industry.

Another group of substances present in some plants is the *tannins*. They are very varied in their chemical composition, but they have some properties in common: they give a blue, green or black colour to anything containing iron, and they have an astringent action. This last property is the basis of their use in medicines.

The delicate smell and flavour of many aromatic plants is due to another type of compound, the *essential oils*. They are commonly used in perfumes and in cookery; medicinally, they serve as stimulants and antiseptics. They may have other substances dissolved in them to form *resins*, as is the case in the pine tree, such a characteristic smell in pine forests. Resins can be solidified and used as expectorants or antiseptics, or they can be semi-liquid, like turpentine. Some contain gums, and are called gum-resins, while those that contain special acids are known as balsams.

Probably the most pharmacologically potent type of

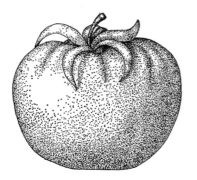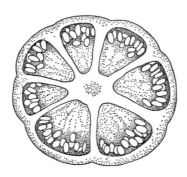

A fleshy fruit, the tomato, seen both whole and in cross section.

substance present in plants is the group of chemicals called *alkaloids.* Morphine, the chief active constituent of opium, is an alkaloid, as is the nicotine of the tobacco plant. Also very powerful are the *glycosides*, which include digitalis, amygdalin, and saponins. The actions of the alkaloids and glycosides are so varied that they cannot be summarized in a few words; they will appear again and again later in the book. Often the bitter substances extracted from plants are either alkaloids (for example, quinine), or glycosides (gentian), although sometimes their detailed composition is uncertain.

Thus, plants contain many different types of chemical compound – we have given only the major ones – and their proportions are very variable, particularly in wild plants. As the plant's biochemistry changes them around, man chooses his moment to harvest and extract the crude drug.

Types of medicine

Having collected the plant, or having obtained a preserved sample containing the active principle, the next step is to extract this activity into a preparation suitable for medicinal use. There are various methods of extraction, and one is chosen according to the ease of extraction of the crude drug and its proposed use.

One of the simplest and best-known types of preparation is the *infusion.* This is made by putting pieces of the dry plant in boiling water, and subsequently straining the water. The procedure is used for chamomile tea – and, indeed for ordinary tea and coffee – and is suitable in cases where the active principle dissolves readily. It is better to mix the herb with boiling water than to boil the mixture; this is a common principle in making coffee, and applies equally well to herbal infusions, where boiling the mixture would destroy or alter the drug.

For a *decoction*, however, this restriction does not apply. This type of preparation is made by putting the plant in cold water, boiling it for 15 to 30 minutes, and then filtering the mixture. The flowers and leaves of mallows, for example, are treated in this way, in order to extract the mucilage for use as a cough remedy.

In making a *macerate*, no heat is used, but the plant is allowed to stand in cold water for a time before the mixture is filtered. An example of a slightly different type of macerate is the misnamed 'quassia infusion': the wood of *Quassia amara* contains bitter substances which dissolve easily in water, and it was once a common practice in Africa to make thick tumblers of this wood. When the tumblers were filled with water, the bitters dissolved to make a drink with eupeptic properties. The tumblers were used over and over again, each time providing a bitter macerate.

A *tincture* is a macerate made not with water, but with alcohol. The dry plant is allowed to stand in the alcohol for several days, after which time the active principles will have dissolved into the solvent. It is a simple means of extracting substances that dissolve more easily in alcohol than in water; gentian tincture is an example.

If a plant is left in any solvent for a while (in water, as if to produce a macerate, or in alcohol or ether), and the solution is later allowed to evaporate, then the concentrated fluid is called an *extract*. It may be a fluid extract or, if greater evaporation is allowed, a soft extract. In some cases, all the solvent is evaporated, leaving a dry extract which can be powdered.

To make a *powder*, either from a dry extract or, more commonly, from the original dried plant tissue, the apparatus used is a pestle and mortar, perhaps the most traditional of all the herbalist's (and pharmacist's) tools. Alternatively, a small mill may be used, but often the long-established method is the more satisfactory. In any case, the plant must be completely dry, which may mean heating it first in an oven, or drying it in air. A pestle and mortar has a crushing action; in a mill the plant is ground. The powder is finally sieved or sifted, to leave only the finest particles.

Pills are made by incorporating powders or extracts in a suitable base, such as starch, glycerin or a gum. The

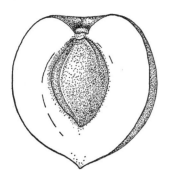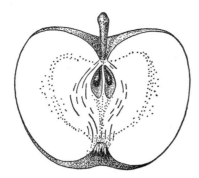

Two more fleshy fruits: the apricot (left) is a drupe fruit; the apple (right) is a pome fruit.

mixture is made into a ball, held together by the filler ingredients, and may be coated. (This is not, in fact, the same thing as a *tablet*. The latter may contain a filling powder, such as starch, as well as the active constituent, but it is made to hold together by being compressed in a machine. In medicine, pills are now almost entirely superseded by tablets, even though we still talk loosely of pills. Even 'The Pill' is really a tablet. The only medicines prepared as true pills are the herbal medicines, such as those described in this book.)

Other means of extracting the medicinal constituents of a plant are by making juices and pulps. *Juices* can be obtained in a number of ways: lemon juice, for example, is extracted simply by pressing the fruit, whereas that of the ash tree is collected by cutting the trunk; after a few hours the juice coagulates into a white mass which is sold as a purgative for children. *Pulp* is made from the soft parts of a plant, without any additions; for this reason pulps easily deteriorate, and have to be made immediately before use. For example, to prepare prune pulp, the dried fruits are soaked in warm water for two hours, the stones removed, and the flesh then pulverized and strained. Finally, the pulp is gently heated until it reaches a uniform consistency. The addition of sugar before heating results in a conserve – jam or jelly.

If a quantity of sugar – which may be up to 75 per cent of the total – is added to a juice, or to an infusion or decoction, the resulting solution is called a *syrup*. The main reason for preparing a syrup is to disguise a disagreeable taste in the medicine.

All the preparations described so far are for internal use, but there are others devised for external application. A *poultice*, for example, is formed from pastes containing oils, starch and mucilages, and may be applied either hot or cold to the skin. Secondly, a *plaster* is a mixture of wax, resins and fats, together with the crude drug; it is placed on a strip of linen and applied to the skin. Finally, a *liniment* is any kind of medicine used externally as an unction or friction, to be applied to the skin or rubbed into the scalp.

How much to take?

When a medicine is prepared into its most suitable form for administration, there remains the question of dosage. This is a vitally important matter, because doses that are too high can cause side-effects, or even death, while doses that are too low or taken at the wrong time may be ineffective. In addition, some drugs can be taken repeatedly, while others have a long-term effect and should be used only for short periods.

It is not possible for anyone but a recognized dispenser of drugs to make a good judgment about dosage. This is particularly true of herbal medicines which, unlike synthetic medicines, are not always of a standard strength. The dose is therefore a matter for the medical practitioner, in the case of medicines controlled by law. For other medicines, particularly those which can be bought over the counter of a shop, the instructions on the packet must be followed with care.

Some of the plants described in this book, however, are readily available for use in the home: examples are food plants such as the rhubarb and the various types of berry. In these cases it is possible to try the effect for oneself, but this should be done with care and in small doses to begin with; or better still, after taking advice.

No doses at all are quoted in this book, even for homely plants such as these. The reason is that methods of preparation inevitably vary, and the plants themselves are not of consistent quality. Thus, to say 'boil and drink one cupful' could result in someone giving himself a uselessly weak dose, roughly the right dose for his needs, or, at worst, a harmful overdose.

Medicinal foods

Many of the plants that we eat for food can be used – in different quantities or recipes – for their pharmacological effect. Indeed, they may exert some effect even when they are taken in the normal way: a drink of coffee is a well-known stimulant, and there are other examples.

11

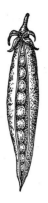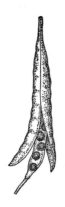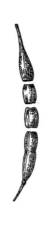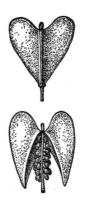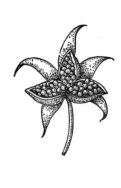

Some dry fruits: pea pod; siliqua (pod) of cabbage; jointed siliqua of radish; silicula (short pod) of shepherd's purse; violet capsule.

Yeast, which in this context can be considered a plant, is one of the favourite 'health foods'. Its major use, both in brewing and baking, is to ferment sugars, forming carbon dioxide and alcohol. Medicinally, however, it is the yeast itself which is of interest, since it is one of the most concentrated known sources of nutriment. Fresh yeast is a yellowish-grey paste, becoming greyish white and crumbly when dry, and consists of millions of micro-organisms – strictly speaking, fungi – of the genus *Saccharomyces*. Yeast is very rich in B vitamins, and has also been recommended specifically for intestinal disorders. In general, it is taken as a regular dose by people who wish to remain in good health, particularly with regard to natural vitamins.

Among the cereals, rice (*Oryza sativa*) can be used medicinally. When it has been boiled for a long time, it is said to be of value in the treatment of colitis and gallstones. Wheat (*Triticum*), when used whole, is a source of vitamins and of wheatgerm oil, and like yeast it is popular as a health food. Also, recent research has shown that whole wheat bread, or other roughage, can prevent certain diseases of the colon which are encouraged by highly refined cereals.

Olive oil (from *Olea europaea*) is said to stimulate the secretion of bile, and also acts as a laxative; it is used to treat intestinal inflammation and for enemas in severe cases of constipation. It can also be applied to scratches and eczema on the skin.

Spinach (*Spinacea oleracea*) is often thought of as a particularly healthy vegetable. It may be effective in cases of weight loss, and is thought to stimulate the pancreatic juices, but it must not be eaten in very large quantities because it contains oxalic acid. Certainly it is not recommended for anyone with a kidney disorder. Nutritionally, it does contain iron, but not in very useful form (contrary to popular opinion). It is, however, an excellent source of vitamin K; this may be the reason why Popeye found it so useful!

The leaves of the rhubarb plant (*Rheum palmatum*) also contain oxalic acid, and are very dangerous, although the rhizomes form a useful laxative, even in the normal quantities taken for food.

The seeds of the marrow (*Cucurbita pepo*) are one of the plant remedies that can be used to remove tapeworms. A purgative has to be taken a few hours afterwards, and the treatment must be repeated two or three times.

The leaves and husks of the walnut (*Juglans regia*) can be made into a decoction with astringent properties, used for alleviating pharyngitis, gastroenteritis accompanied by diarrhea, conjunctivitis and dermatitis.

Among the spices, black mustard seeds (*Sinapis nigra*) can be made into a soothing poultice which is thought to alleviate muscular pain, rheumatism, arthritis, bronchitis and pneumonia. The same seeds can be used in sauces, but for cooking it is usually preferable to use white mustard seeds (*Sinapis alba*), whose effect is similar to that of black mustard seeds, but is milder. The flower heads of basil (*Ocimum basilicum*) are used to prepare a mouthwash, and to treat weeping wounds.

These are just a few examples of the various kinds of food plants – vegetables, herbs and spices – which can be used medicinally as well as for their taste or nutritive value. Many more examples are included in the illustrations later in the book.

Wild and exotic plants

Most plants that are used for their medicinal properties are not edible, in the usual sense of the word; indeed, some can be quite poisonous. They include wild flowers, trees, ornamental plants, exotic plants – almost every kind of vegetation is represented one way or another in medicinal remedies.

Among the ornamental plants, for example, is the cypress tree, in particular *Cupressus sempervirens*, whose cones contain substances that are useful in the treatment of diseases of the circulatory system: hemorrhoids (piles), varicose veins, and so on. The mistletoe (*Viscum album*), a semi-parasitic plant found on fruit and conifer trees, is another example. Its leaves and young shoots can be

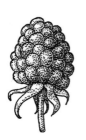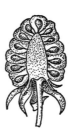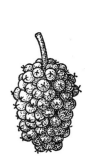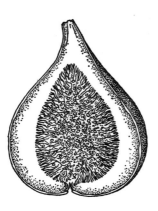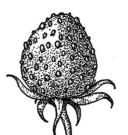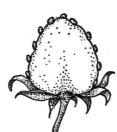

Some false fruits: blackberry, whole and in section; mulberry; fig, in section; strawberry, whole and in section.

prepared and used to reduce blood pressure. Again, the flowering shoots of the passion flower (*Passiflora incarnata*) make a useful medicament with a tranquillizing action. The rhizome of the butcher's broom (*Ruscus aculeatus*) is used to make a diuretic and aperient concoction. And the leaves of another ornamental plant, the laurel (*Laurus nobilis*), can be made into a decoction, with the addition of orange peel, for the treatment of some types of gastric and rheumatic complaints.

Many exotic plants are famous for their medicinal properties. Indeed, one of the best known of all healing plants is the cinchona (*Cinchona calisaya*), from which quinine is obtained, and this is an exotic species. It is native to Peru and northern Bolivia, and is also grown in Java and Ceylon. The plant was named by Linnaeus after the Countess of Chinchon (wife of the Viceroy of Peru) who had reputedly been cured of malaria by cinchona bark, and who subsequently distributed it to the poor. It is of interest that quinine is still important today, particularly when the malaria parasite becomes resistant to synthetic drugs, as among American troops in Vietnam. Cinchona is a good example of how a plant medicine can suffer the setbacks and favours of history; between its auspicious start and its present popularity, it was at one time restricted in use because of religious opposition to the Jesuits who introduced it to Europe.

Other exotic species of importance include the senna (*Cassia fistula*), a tree cultivated in tropical regions for its purgative properties; the tamarind (*Tamarindus indica*), another tropical tree of which the fruit-pulp is thirst-quenching and laxative; and *Strophanthus kombe*, which provides the glycoside called strophanthin. This climbing tree grows in East Africa, and the drug it yields has found an established place in therapeutics because of its action on the heart. As a final example, one of the most exotic-sounding species is in fact not quite as romantic as it sounds: gum arabic comes not from Arabia at all, but from an African species, *Acacia senegal*. It is used as a gum and also in the form of a syrup, for pharyngitis and gastroenteritis.

Not just for drugs

Just as some plants that are chiefly grown for food or ornamental purposes can be a source of drugs, so a number of primarily or potentially medicinal plants are put to other uses by man, in his ingenious attempts to utilize all natural resources to their fullest advantage. For example, plants that are used for textile fibres (for example, flax), for religious purposes (incense), or, in many cases, for personal pleasure (tobacco, lavender perfume, and so on), have potential medicinal uses that are not generally known or are ignored by most people.

To give a rather different example, the camphor tree is known for its medicinal uses, but camphor – the distillation product of the wood and leaves – is now of industrial importance. Indeed, it can now be produced synthetically, although at one time the tree was the only source, and it retains its value as an insecticide (particularly against the clothes moth), and as a starting material in the synthesis of celluloid and varnishes.

The medicinal use of flax (*Linum usitatissum*), already mentioned, is in poultices for respiratory ailments, while another textile plant, cotton (*Gossypium herbaceum*), is almost as valuable in the preparation of cotton-wool and gauze dressings as it is in shirts and dresses. In addition, an edible oil can be extracted from the seeds.

Finally, the gifts of the Magi are not without their healing properties. Incense, already mentioned, is a gum-resin obtained from the bark of *Boswellia carteri*, a tree found mainly in Arabia and Somalia. Besides its religious use, it may be used for fumigation in cases of respiratory infection, and in plasters for rheumatism. Myrrh is also a gum-resin, from the bark of *Commiphora abyssinica*, a tree that grows in Abyssinia. It can be used as a mouthwash in the treatment of gingivitis and pyorrhea, or even in toothpaste.

Having talked of incense and myrrh, it would be a pity not to mention the gift of the third Wise Man, even though it was not from a plant: gold is used in the treatment of rheumatic disorders, as well as for filling teeth!

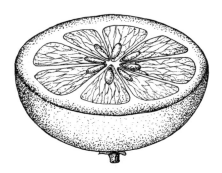 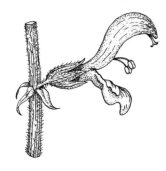

Left: Section through a bitter orange, a hesperidium fruit. Right: The bilabiate (two-lipped) appearance of the sage flower.

Summary

Finally, let us summarize the purpose of this book, and the use that can be made of it. It is, we hope, at the least a collection of clear photographs of some important medicinal plants, with a description of how each one can be of value to man. Our attempt is not to provide a comprehensive guide to the practice of herbal medicine: that would be barely possible, and certainly dangerous, in view of the wide variation in plant species in different areas. But the information here should be of interest and help to anyone who prefers herbal to conventional medicine, and should at the same time illustrate how important are the natural, medicinal species to the modern drug empires. Not only does industry continue to extract crude drugs from many species of plants; but also, a considerable number of the drugs that are now artificially synthesized are based on man's experience with natural compounds, and are in some cases an imitation of Nature, standardized and mass-produced in factories all over the world.

Above all, we hope to show that among the many beautiful plants of the world, and, indeed, the plain ones too, are some that have surprising power over our bodies; botanical factories of intricate chemical compounds, for man to pluck and use for his health.

Bibliography

Most of the ancient herbals are now available only in libraries and museums, and are worth looking at if one has the opportunity. Some, like Culpeper's, have been edited and reissued. There are many other books on the subject; the selection given here should provide further reading for anyone interested in medicinal plants.

Chopra, R. N., *Glossary of Indian medicinal plants*, Pergamon Press, Oxford 1956

Claus, E. P., Taylor, V. E., and Brady, L. R., *Pharmacognosy*, 6th edition, Lea & Febiger, Philadelphia 1970

Ferguson, N. M., *A textbook of pharmacognosy*, Macmillan, New York 1956

Hocking, G. M., *A dictionary of terms in pharmacognosy*, Blackwell, Oxford, and Charles C. Thomas, Illinois, 1955

Kreig, M. B., *Green medicine*, Harrap, London 1965

Leyer, C. F. (ed.), *Culpeper's English physician and complete herbal*, Arco, London 1961

Taylor, N., *Plant drugs that changed the world*, Dodd, Mead & Co., New York 1965

Todd, R. G. (ed.), *Extra Pharmacopoeia (Martindale)*, 25th edition, Pharmaceutical Press, London 1967

Trease, G. E., and Evans, W. C., *Pharmacognosy*, 10th edition, Baillière Tindall, London 1972

Watt, J. M., and Breyer-Brandwijk, M. G., *The medicinal and poisonous plants of southern and eastern Africa*, 2nd edition, Livingstone, Edinburgh and London 1962

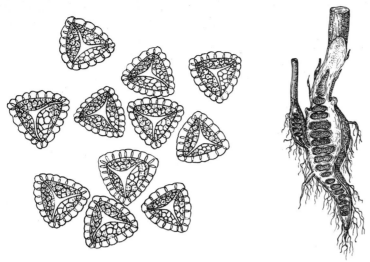

Left. Spores may help in identification; these are from lycopodium.
Right: an aquatic type of root, from the hemlock plant.

Glossary of terms

Active principle. The chemical component of a crude drug which has a therapeutic effect

Alkaloid. A type of complex organic chemical which occurs naturally in plants

Antiseptic. A substance that inhibits the growth of bacteria

Antispasmodic. A substance that relieves a muscular spasm

Aperitive. Stimulating the appetite

Astringent. A substance that shrinks tissues and prevents the secretion of fluids

Bulbs. Modified plant buds, with scale leaves, which occur beneath the soil

Calyx. The outermost envelope of the flower, consisting of a number of sepals

Carminative. A substance that relieves flatulence

Cathartic. Strongly laxative

Conjunctivitis. Inflammation of the front of the eye

Corolla. The petals of a flower

Cystitis. Infection of the bladder and urinary tract

Deciduous. Seasonal and simultaneous shedding of leaves

Decoction. An extract of a crude drug obtained by boiling in water

Dehiscent. Describes a fruit which splits open when ripe

Demulcent. A soothing medicine

Depurative. A purifying agent, normally applied to blood purifying agents

Dermatitis. Inflammation of the skin

Diaphoretic. A substance for increasing perspiration

Diuretic. A substance that helps the body to dispose of water, by increasing the amount of urine produced

Drupe. A fleshy fruit with a hard stone, such as a plum

Eczema. An inflammatory disease of the skin

Emetic. A substance that causes vomiting

Emmenagogue. A substance that brings on menstruation

Emollient. A preparation for softening tissues

Enema. Any liquid preparation introduced into the rectum

Eupeptic. A substance that promotes good digestion

Expectorant. A substance that promotes the ejection of fluid from the lungs and trachea

Gastroenteritis. Inflammation of the stomach and intestine, characterized by pain, nausea and diarrhea

Gingivitis. Inflammation of the gums

Glycosides. A type of chemical found in plants

Gum. A viscous fluid exuded by some plants which discolours and hardens on exposure to air and light

Hemostatic. A substance which prevents bleeding and promotes clotting

Indehiscent. Fruits which remain closed on reaching maturity

Inflorescence. The flowerhead of a plant

Infusion. The solution produced by adding hot water to part of a plant

Latex. A milky juice produced by certain plants

Laxative. A substance that encourages defecation

Macerate. A cold-water extract of a plant

Mucilage. A gum-like material produced by some plants

Peduncle. The stalk attached to a flower

Pharmacognosy. The study of the biology, chemistry and pharmacology of plant drugs, herbs and spices

Pharmacology. The study of the actions of chemicals and drugs in the body

Pharmacy. The preparation and dispensing of drugs

Pharyngitis. Inflammation of the throat

Psoriasis. A skin disease

Pulmonary. Concerned with the lungs

Purgative. A powerful laxative

Pyorrhea. A discharge of pus from the gums and teeth

Rhizome. An underground stem

Saponin. A plant glycoside which foams in water

Sepal. A segment of the calyx

Stimulant. A substance that stimulates activity of the body

Stomachic. An agent that promotes activity of the stomach

Stomatitis. Inflammation of the mouth

Tannins. A group of astringent plant constituents

Therapeutics. The branch of medicine associated with the use of remedies and the treatment of diseases

Tincture. An alcoholic extract of a plant drug

Tuber. A swollen underground stem, *eg* potato

Umbel. An umbrella-shaped inflorescence

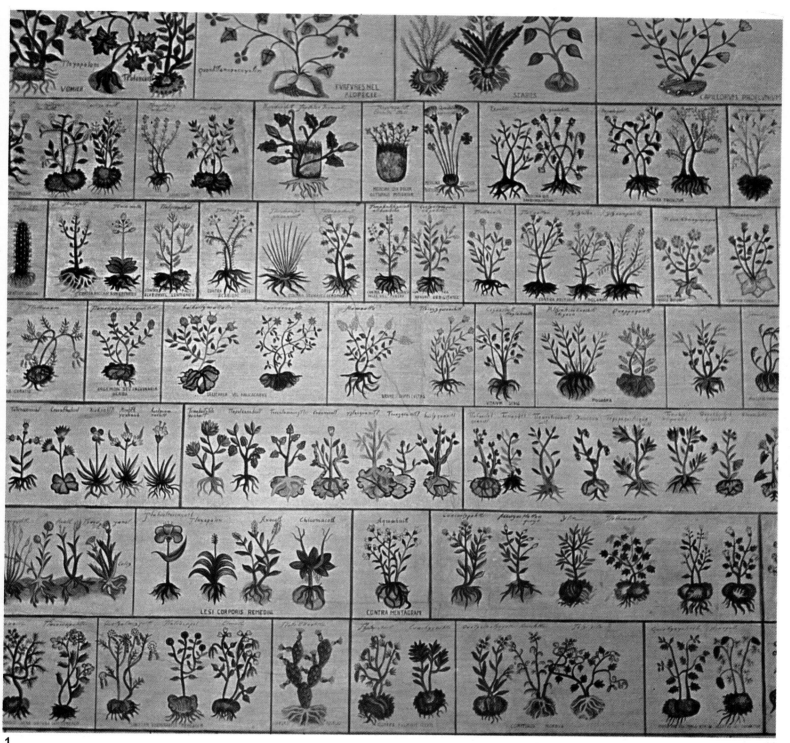

1 This wall painting by the modern Mexican artist Diego Rivera is copied from a fourteenth-century Aztec codex. Detailed drawings of this kind were valuable in the Middle Ages, when herbal medicines formed the basis of all therapies. Written descriptions could explain the use of the plants, but could not help as much as drawings in precise identification. The mural can be seen on the wall of the National School of Agriculture, near Mexico City.

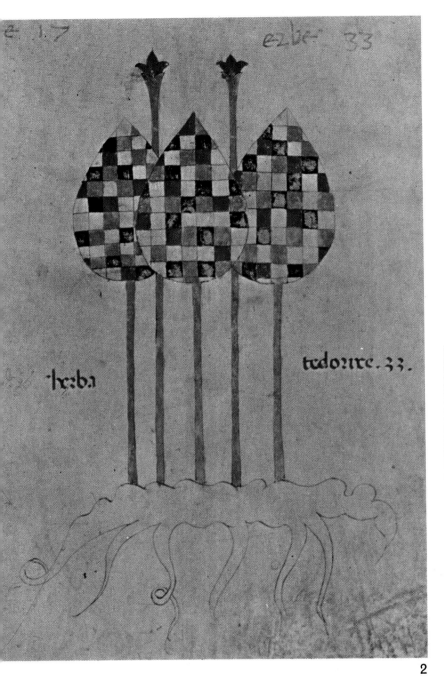

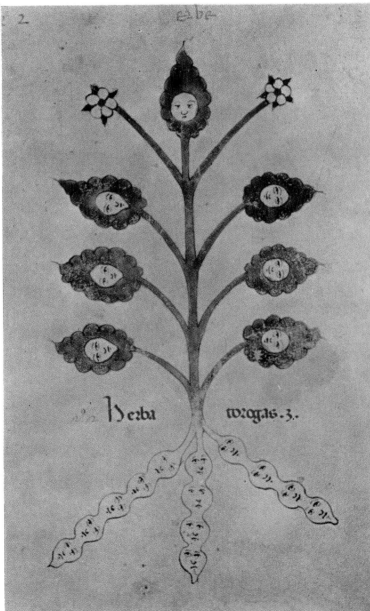

2–3 These two illustrations, taken from a medieval herbal, show that the artists of the day were not always concerned with accurate and informative detail, but used their imagination to devise fanciful species with interesting – though often fictional – properties. Many authors of the time used for reference the very earliest book of medicinal plants, written in the first century BC by the Greek doctor Crateva, and kept in Byzantium until the sixteenth century.

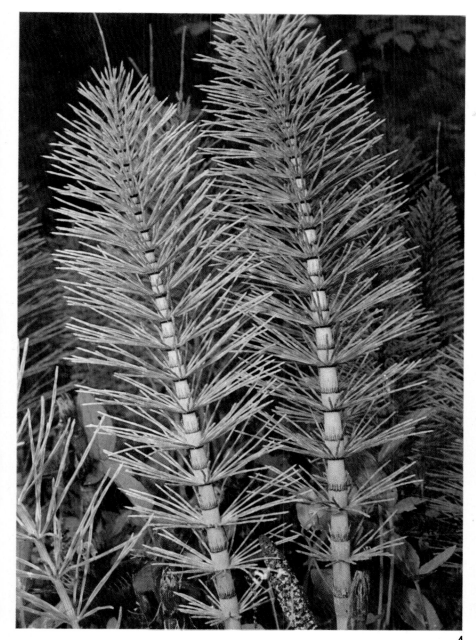

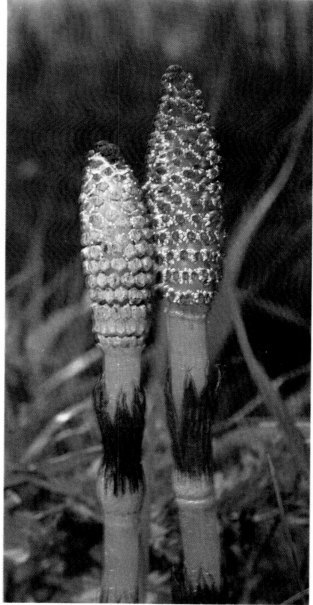

4-5 The horsetail (*Equisetum telmateia*) may carry either sterile shoots or fertile shoots. The green, sterile shoots have a weak diuretic action, and this is the plant's only modern use. In the past, however, along with a score of other horsetail species, particularly *E. arvense*, it was recommended for tuberculosis.

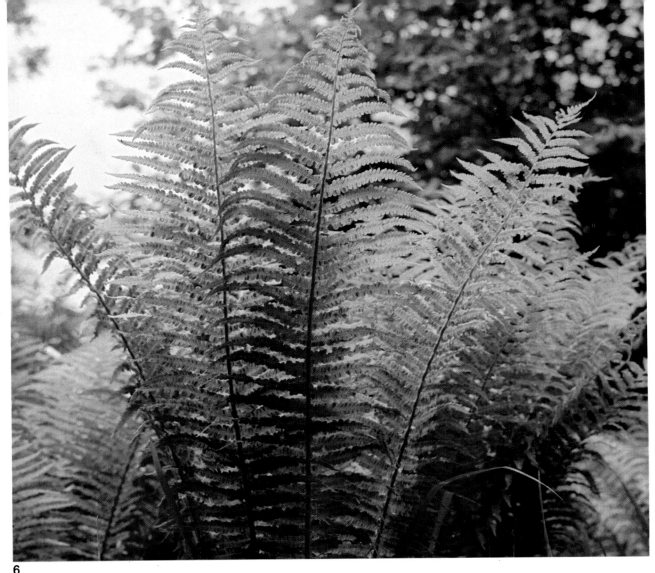

6

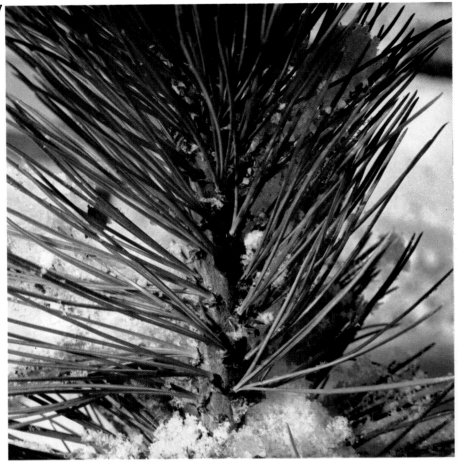

7

6 The male fern (*Dryopteris felix-mas*) contains a substance called filicin, which is effective against intestinal worms. The active agent is extracted, using ether from the rhizomes, frond bases and buds, and is available in capsule form in many countries. The fern extract is not safe for elderly, debilitated or pregnant patients, and, when used, should be followed by a mild purgative.

7 There are many species of pine – approaching a hundred – and most have been of some use as medicines. They provide turpentine and colcophony, for example, as well as other oils and resins used in ointments. Illustrated here is *Pinus cembra*, the arolla pine, which grows in mountainous regions and has edible seeds.

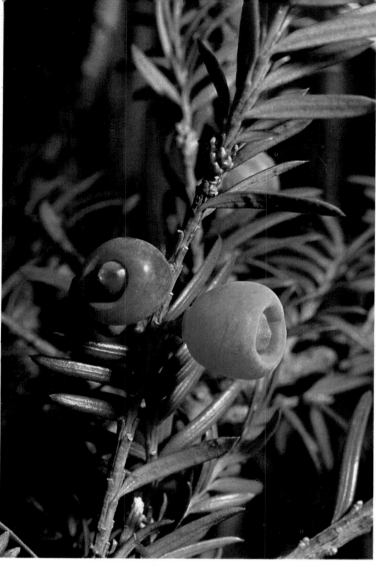

8 The yew tree (*Taxus baccata*) is included here as a warning: it is deadly poisonous. This applies to all parts of the tree, even those which appear in ancient herbals as cures for one thing or another. Its delicate pink seeds and dark green leaves have tempted many animals, and children too, with tragic consequences.

9 This type of juniper tree (*Juniperus oxycedra*) is a source of cade oil, once an important treatment of some skin conditions, particularly psoriasis, but now superseded in this by coal tar ointments. Juniper tar oil is still featured in modern pharmacopeias, and is used as a local cure in Mediterranean regions where this tree, the prickly juniper, grows.

10 *Arum maculatum*, commonly called cuckoo-pint or lords-and-ladies, is a very poisonous plant, particularly when fresh. Nevertheless, its starchy tubers can be a source of food, and tinctures prepared from both the leaves and the tubers have been used in the treatment of conditions affecting digestion, respiration, and the joints.

10

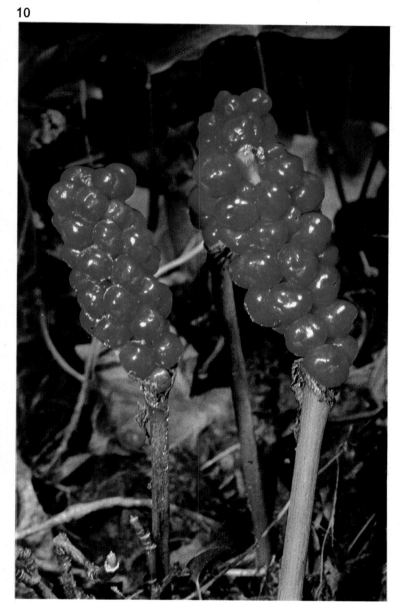

8

9

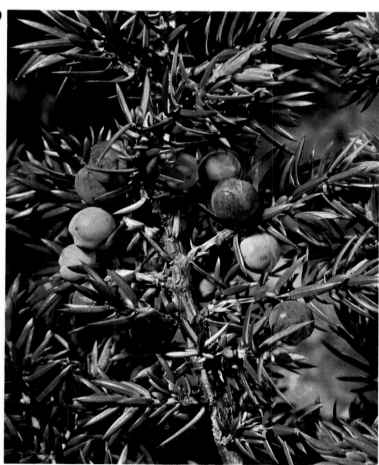

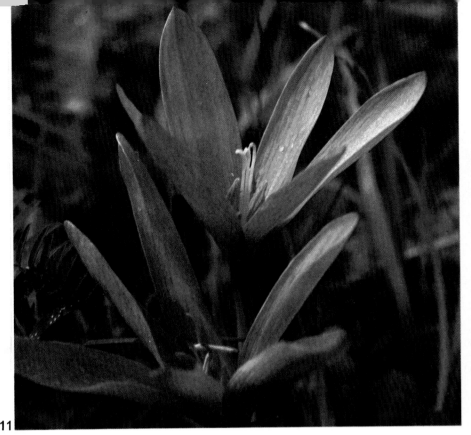

11

12

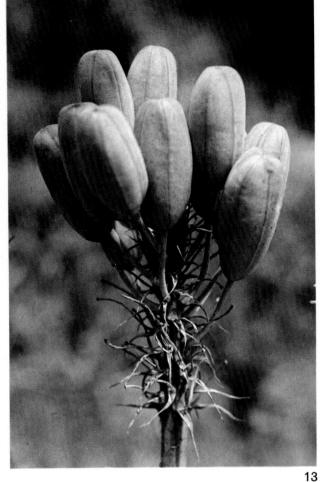

13

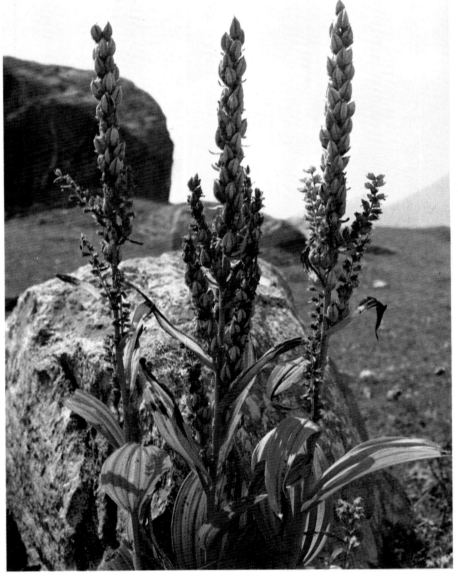

11 The autumn crocus (*Colchicum autumnale*) is a source of a substance called colchicine, which is important for two reasons. First, it has a long history in the treatment of gout, and, indeed, is still used for this purpose today. Secondly, it is a powerful inhibitor of cell-division, and is therefore of great value in many areas of research in such subjects as genetics and cytology. The plant is highly poisonous, and should not be used as a herbal remedy in any form.

12 The white hellebore (*Veretrum album*) is a source of a mixture of alkaloids known generally as veratrine, which can reduce blood pressure. It is no longer used, however, because of its unpleasant side-effects, and when veratrine preparations are required the green hellebore is a rather safer source.

13 There are many species of *Aloe*, all of them native to hot, arid regions, and now widely grown for ornamental purposes. They have a capsule-like fruit (shown here), but it is the fleshy leaves that have a pharmacological action: when cut, they exude a liquid which dries to give a bitter-tasting purgative.

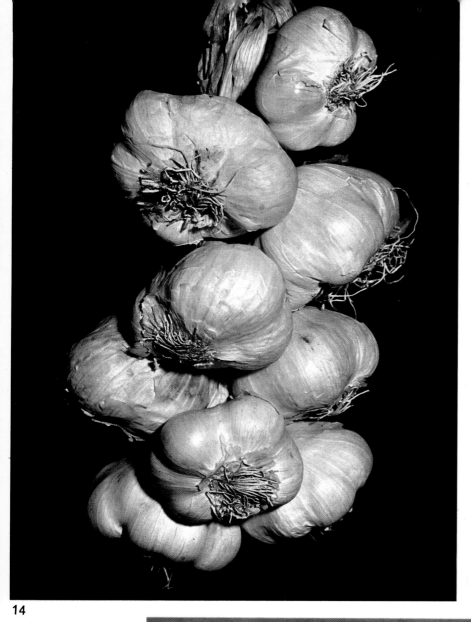

14 Cloves of garlic (*Allium sativum*) are a familiar sight in kitchens, and they can also be used medicinally. Apart from being a potent antiseptic, garlic is excellent for colds, influenza and bronchitis, because of its expectorant and diaphoretic properties. It should be emphasized, however, that preparations of garlic – aside from the very small amounts used in cooking – are dangerous to children.

15 The onion (*Allium capa*) has had various therapeutic properties claimed for it: examples are the cure of anemia, reduction of blood pressure, and antibacterial actions. Its main herbal uses, however, are as a diuretic and to alleviate intestinal discomfort. Recently, doctors have found evidence that onion helps to keep down the amount of fat in the blood circulation, which may make it useful in the control of heart disease; interestingly, the French have for centuries given both onion and garlic to their horses to cure them of similar circulatory complaints.

14

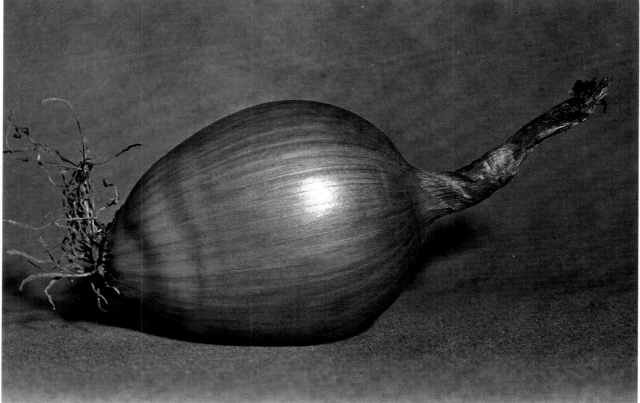

15

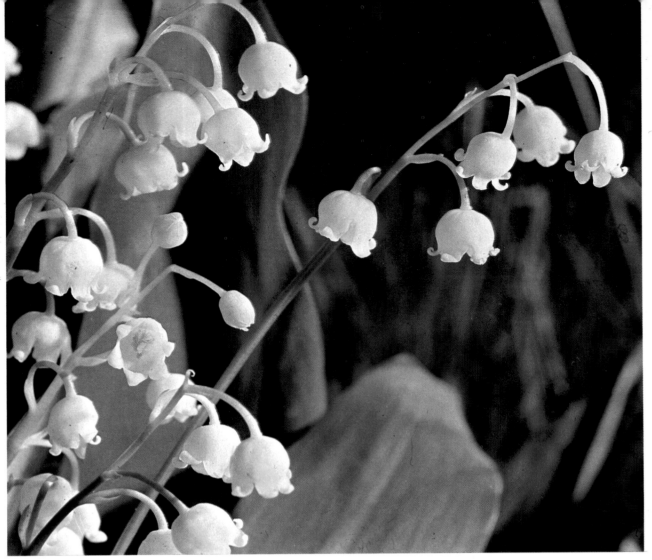

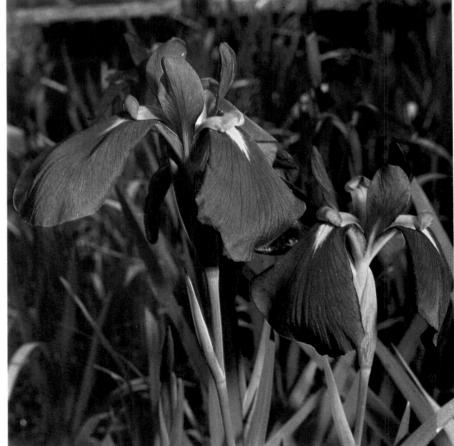

16 The roots and, to a lesser extent, the flowers of the lily of the valley (*Convallaria majalis*) can be dried and ground into a powder, or made into an infusion, which has the same beneficial effect on a weak heart as does digitalis, which is obtained from foxgloves.

17 This is an example of the genus *Iris*, some of whose species have medicinal properties, having been used in toothpastes and dusting powders. The dried rhizome is the source of the active agent, which is mainly used now as a base for cosmetics, particularly violet perfumes.

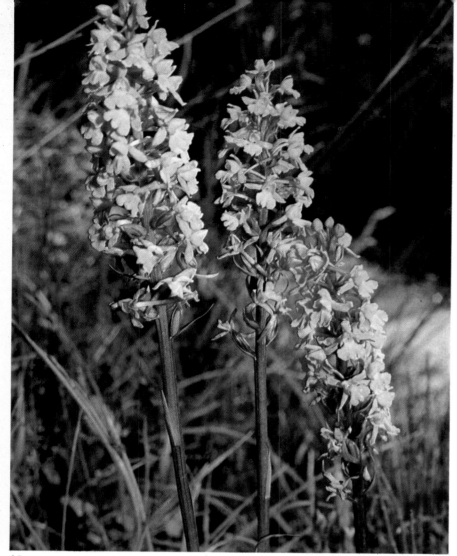

18

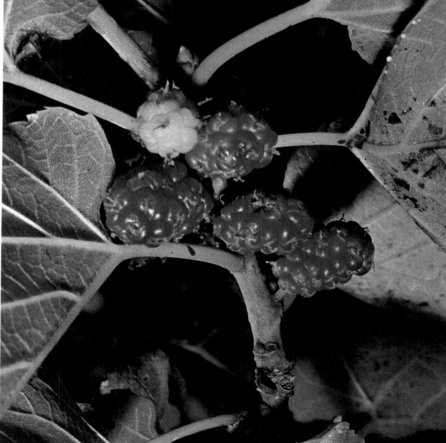

19

18 A popular drink in some parts of Europe is salep, made from the tubers of the early purple orchid (*Orchis mascula*). It is nutritive, since the tubers contain starch, and it also has soothing properties, allaying irritation of the stomach and intestine.

19 The juice obtained from mulberries (*Morus nigra*), made into a syrup with sugar, has been used as an expectorant. It also has a slight laxative effect, and has been used in various conditions as an astringent. With this plant there is little danger of poisoning, as it is widely eaten anyway as a fruit, although too many berries may have too loosening an action.

20 Although this flowering plant may not be immediately recognized, it is in fact one of the best known of all. Its name is *Ricinus communis*, the castor oil plant. The seeds themselves are poisonous in the natural state, or if prepared wrongly, but when the oil is extracted from them and treated, it is a valuable mild purgative. It is also used as a base for some eye ointments, and for emollients, such as zinc and castor oil cream.

21 The inner part of the bark of cinnamon (*Cinnamomum zeylonicum*) is dried and made into a powder or tincture to counteract flatulence. It may also be used to treat diarrhea, because of its astringent nature, but has the disadvantage of causing rectal burning.

22 Most of the numerous species of *Anemone* have pharmacological actions, although they are rather poisonous. Among them are *A. pulsatilla*, popular for menstrual disorders, and *A. hepatica*, a herbal remedy for coughs and chest ailments.

23 A grandiose example of one type of rhubarb (*Rheum palmatum*). This and other species of *Rheum* have cathartic properties; a fact that is known to most people who have over-indulged in rhubarb. Medicinally, a purgative is prepared from the rhizome – the underground part of the stem – and has an astringency which separates it from other, similar purgatives. Indeed, it has been used in the treatment of diarrhea, the idea being that it first clears the bowel and then 'closes' it. Today, however, it is used exclusively as a purgative, and then only for acute, not chronic, constipation.

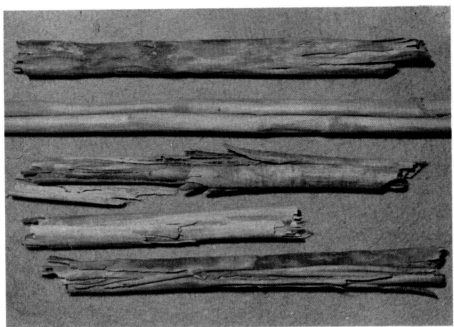

21

20

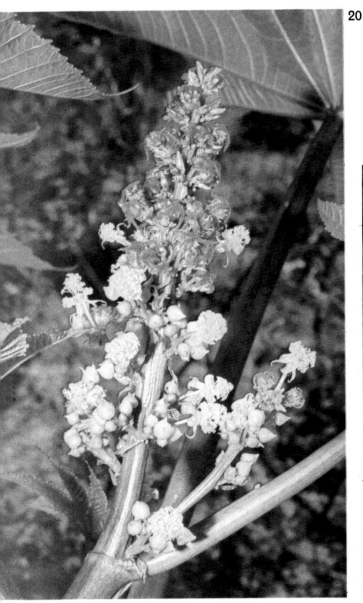

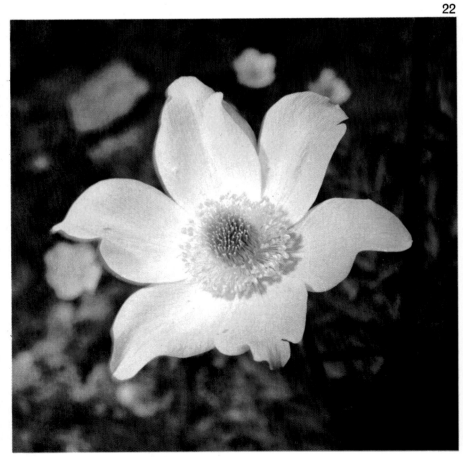

22

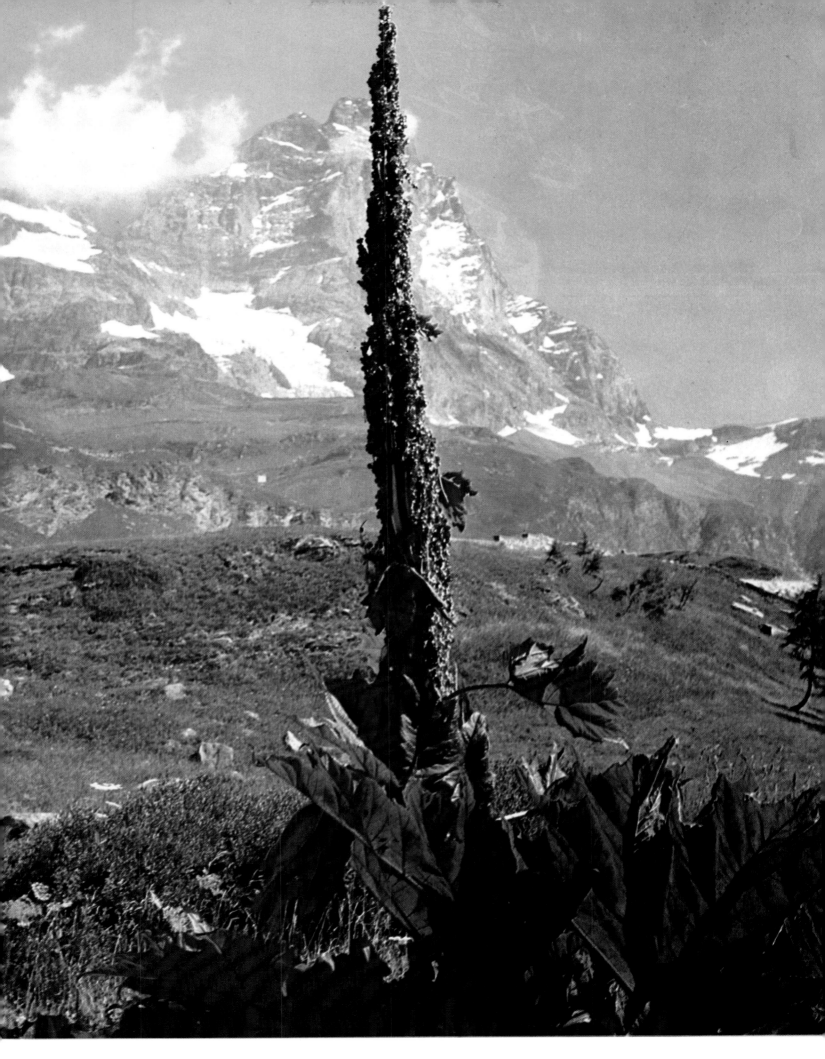

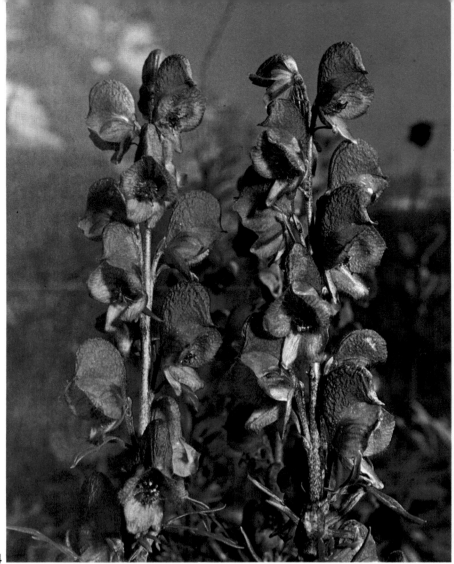

24

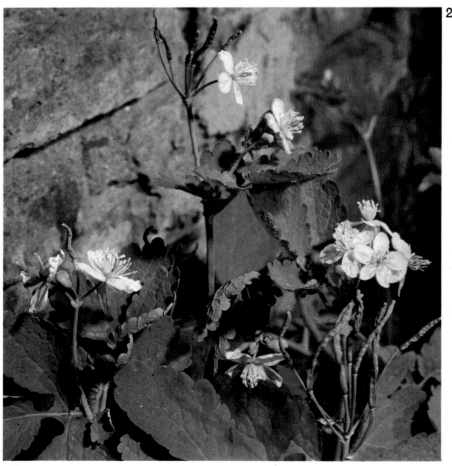

25

24 The monkshood (*Aconitum napellus*) is not common in the wild, but is cultivated for its medicinal properties. It is also known as aconite, and there are several related species which also yield active preparations. The main use of monkshood is in reducing fever, but it is a fairly dangerous remedy since side-effects of toxicity arise all too readily. Applied to the skin – for example in a liniment – it first produces a tingling sensation, and then numbness, and has been used in this way to alleviate rheumatic pains.

25 'Comfort have thou of thy merit,' said Wordsworth in his poem to the celandine; but he was probably not referring to the sedative, expectorant, diuretic and purgative properties of this species, *Chelidonium majus*. The active principle is contained in the orange latex, obtainable from the cut roots.

26 The field poppy (*Papaver rhoeas*) is still occasionally used in the form of a syrup made from the petals, for colouring and sweetening, but the sedative and soothing infusion that can be made from the heads of the plant is now rarely available.

27–28 One of the most valuable, and most widely abused, of all medicinal plants is the opium poppy (*Papaver somniferum*). It originated in the East, where its use as a narcotic drug has a long history; today, it grows wild and in cultivation all over the world. Extraction of the drug is achieved by making transverse cuts in the unripe capsules. The latex that exudes from the incisions contains many alkaloids, of which the most important is morphine; this substance, like its derivative, heroin and opium itself, is very highly addictive and dangerous, as is made clear by the numerous tragic cases in the East and, increasingly, in the civilized countries of North America and Europe. The abuse of these 'hard' drugs, however, does not detract from their enormous value in conventional medicine: morphine is extremely effective against severe pain, and is invaluable in many kinds of emergency.

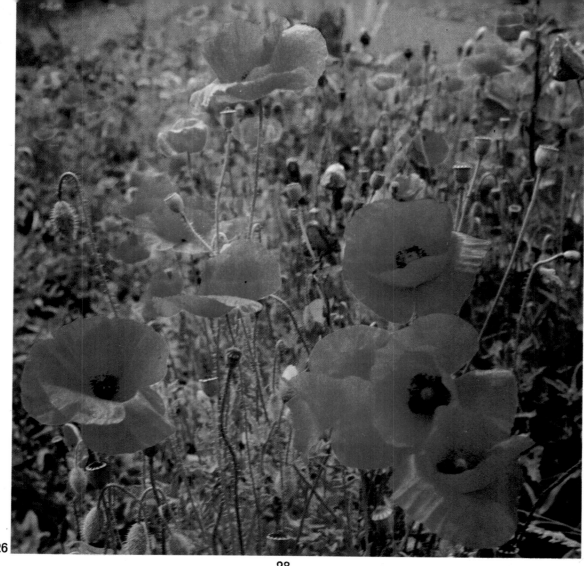

26

27

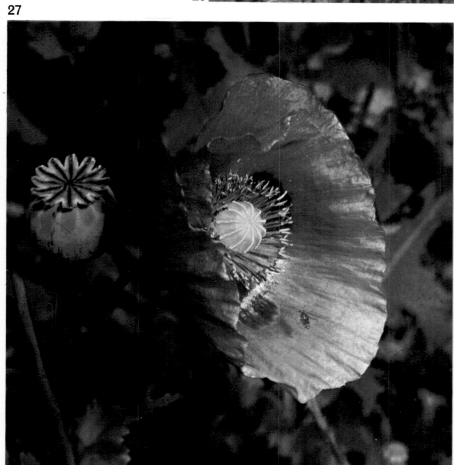

28

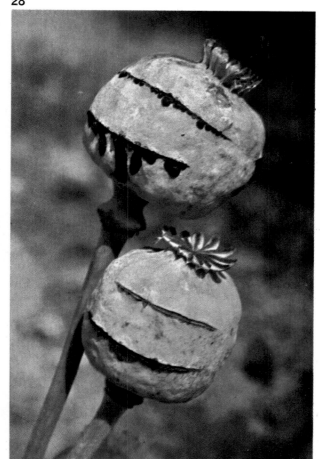

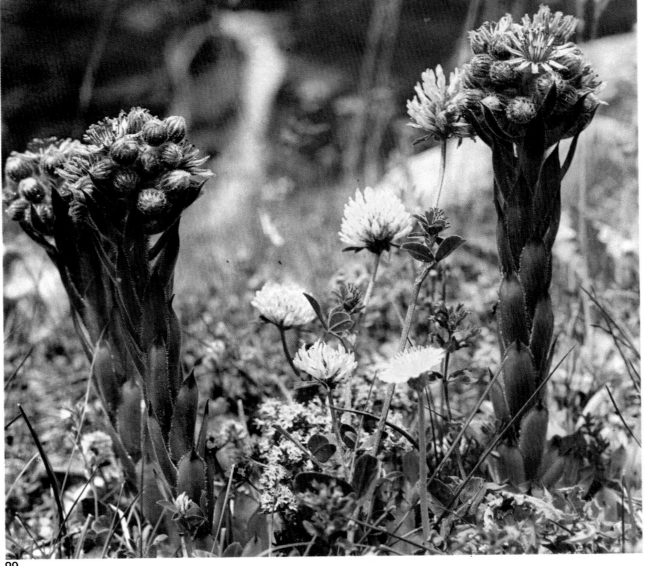

29

30

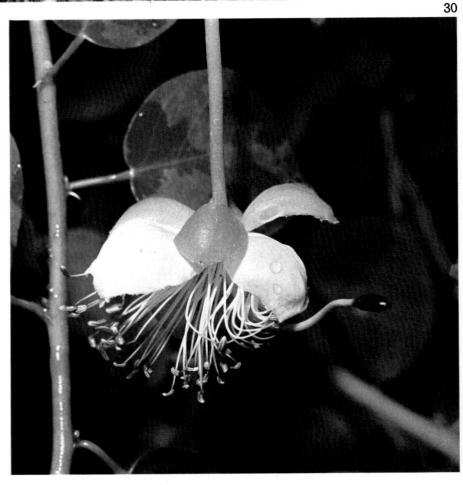

29 *Sempervivum montanum*, the mountain houseleek, is found on the rocks and stones of mountain pastures. Its leaves are used in the preparation of poultices for the healing of burns, insect bites and skin ulcers, while an infusion of the leaves is used as an eye-salve in cases of conjunctivitis. Both the juice and the macerate of the leaves are said to be refreshing and astringent.

30 The beautiful caper plant (*Capparis spinosa*) is best known for its culinary use: the flavouring called 'capers' is made by cooking and pickling the flowerheads. Other preparations from the same plant, particularly of its bark, have featured in herbals but are now rarely heard of.

31 The cobweb houseleek, *Sempervivum arachnoideum*, is found in the same locations as *S. montanum* (see 29), and has much the same herbal properties. It is also cultivated as a pot plant.

32 This is the blackberry (*Rubus fruticosus*), well known and loved as a fruit. The ripe, aggregate berries are a rich source of vitamin C, and, in large amounts, have a purgative action. The leaves are astringent.

33 Another popular fruit is the redcurrant (*Ribes rubrum*), from which syrups, jellies and refreshing drinks are made. It is also used as a flavouring and colouring agent.

34 *Rosa gallica*, a South-European type of wild rose, is the basis of a gargle for soothing an inflamed throat. It is prepared from the distilled essence of the flowers, which is also used in perfumery. Other species of wild rose have been used similarly.

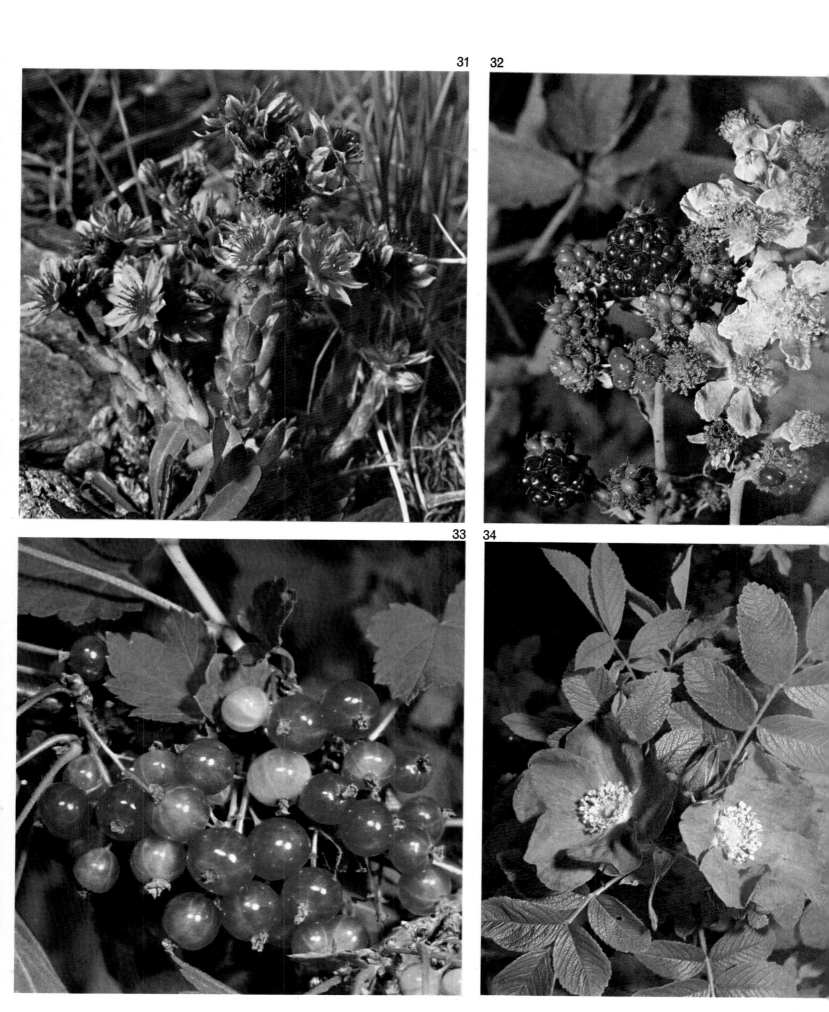

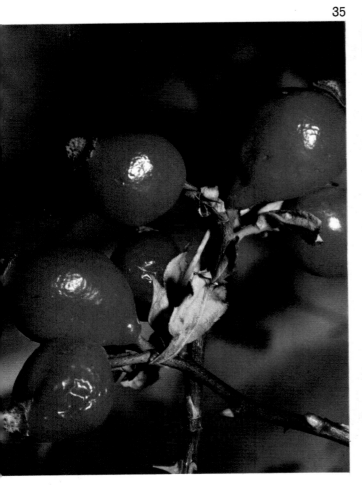

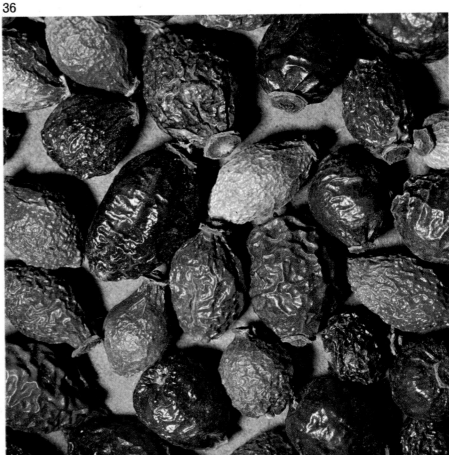

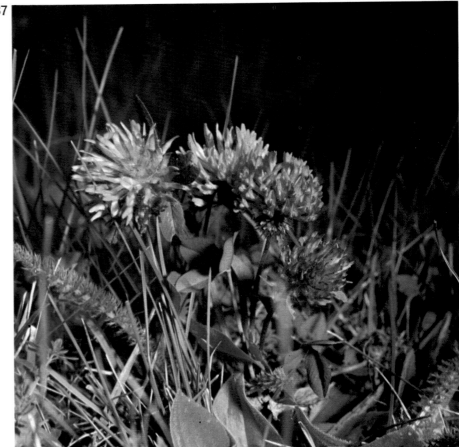

35–36 The fruits of the wild rose (*Rosa gallica, R. canina,* etc.) are called rose hips, and are a very rich source of vitamin C. Rose-hip syrup is one of the most popular vitamin supplements for infants.

37 The red clover (*Trifolium pratense*) is one of the pasture plants of great value to farmers. As a herbal, it is mildly antispasmodic and expectorant, but its main use in medicine is in the treatment of skin conditions, for example chronic eczema. It has also been used in the treatment of whooping cough, but is not used so much today, since this disease is well controlled by vaccination in most countries.

38 The medicinal properties of the rose were recorded in the 'Theatrum Sanitatis' at the end of the fourth century AD. This is one of the illustrations in that book, which is at present kept in the Biblioteca Casanatense, in Rome.

Roxe.

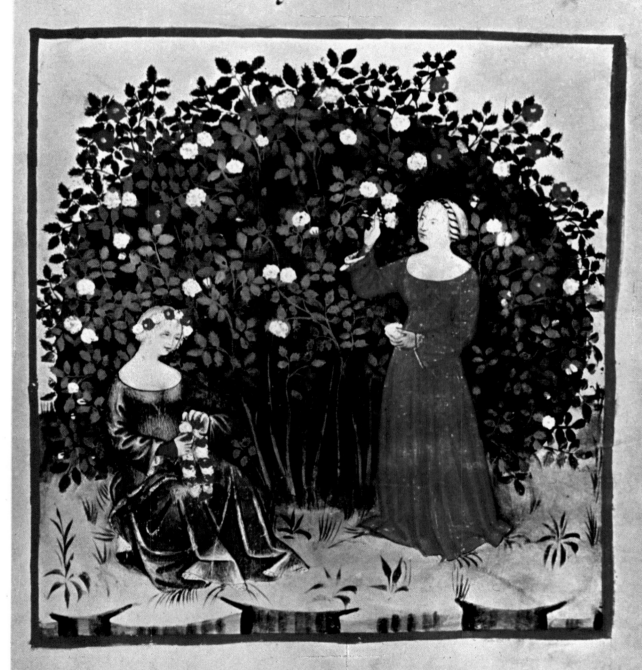

hature f. m 2°. f. m 2. melioz ex eis . de uin y pfia Junamentur. ce
rebzo calido Nocumentu. efficit quibozz mischine. Remoctio nocu
menti . cu camphoza .

·i· soela

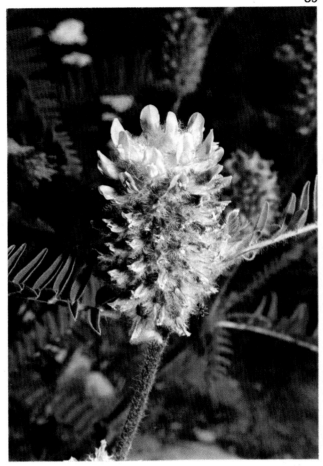

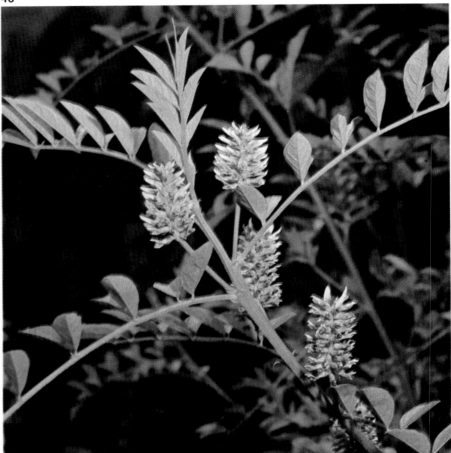

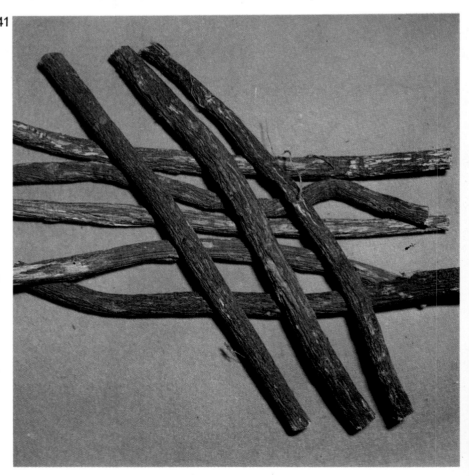

39 Milk vetch is the common name for many species of the genus
Astragalus, for example *A. alopecuroides* (shown here) and
A. gummifer, the main source of gum tragacanth. This valuable gum,
obtainable also from other species of the same genus, is used
widely in both medicine and the food industry as a binder or filler,
and as a mouthwash. Another species, *A. crotalaria*, is called the
'loco weed' in California, Nebraska and Texas. It is poisonous to
cattle, horses and other animals, causing a kind of spinal paralysis.

40–41 The plant *Glycerrhiza glabra* is useful for its rhizomes which
are commonly known as liquorice sticks. When dried or boiled,
liquorice is a source of several important drugs, all chemically
similar. They and their modern synthetic derivatives (such as
carbenoxolone) are extremely valuable in the treatment of gastric
ulcers, and, in some cases, as anti-inflammatory agents.

42 The rue (*Ruta graveolans*), despite its disagreeable smell, is a
powerful herbal, having been widely used in the past – and still today
– as a carminative, antispasmodic and emmenagogue. For these
purposes, it is gathered and prepared into oil of rue during the
flowering season, or used as the dry herb.

43 One of the group of mallows, *Malva sylvestris*, is collected both
for its leaves and its flowers. They are prepared into a domestic
cough remedy because of their demulcent and emollient action,
which is due to the large amount of mucilage in the plant.

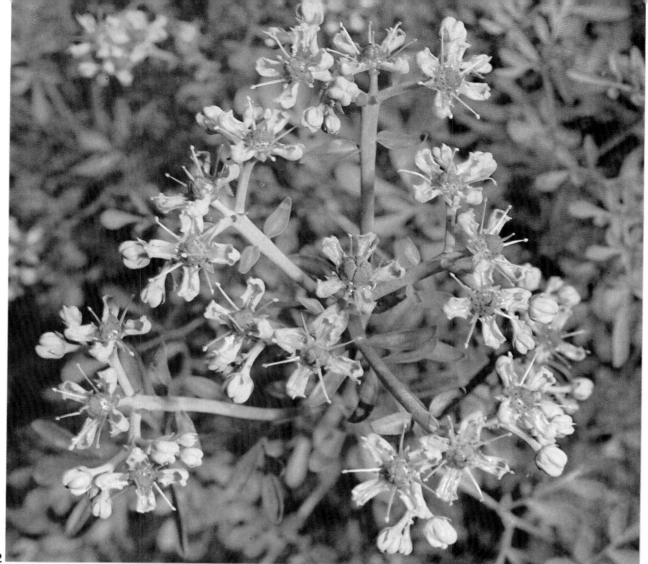

42

43

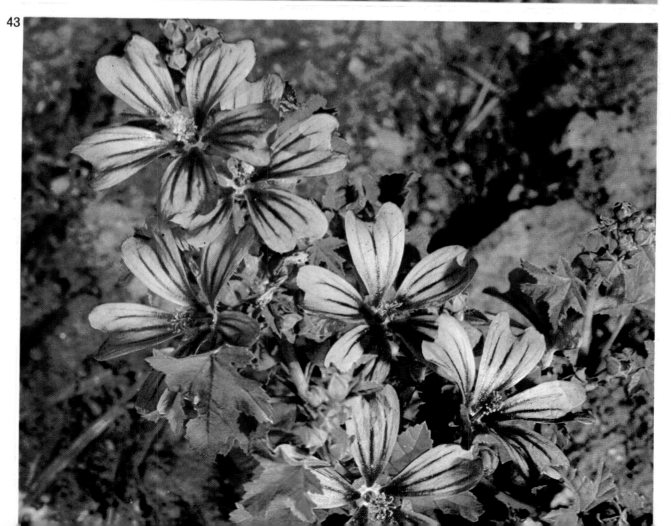

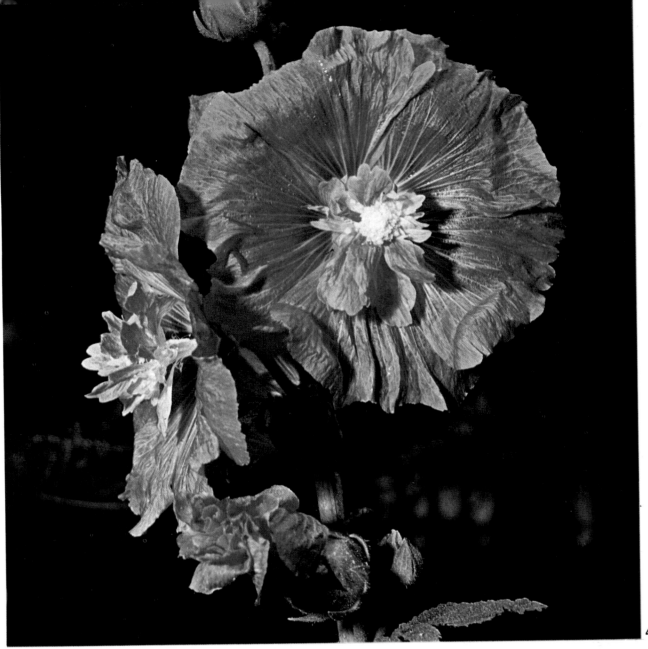

44 The flowers and leaves of the hollyhock, (*Althaea rosea*), a plant often cultivated for its considerable beauty, provide an extract with similar properties to those of the mallow, being used to soothe inflammation of the mouth and throat.

45 The lime tree (*Tilia x. europaea*) is often cultivated by the roadside because it grows quickly and has a long life. Its yellowish leaves may be prepared into a decoction to soothe a sore throat or mouth. It also has a diaphoretic and antispasmodic effect, and is therefore used in colds and for stomach cramp. Lime tea is an established traditional herbal remedy. This is not the same lime tree as the one that provides the citrus fruit.

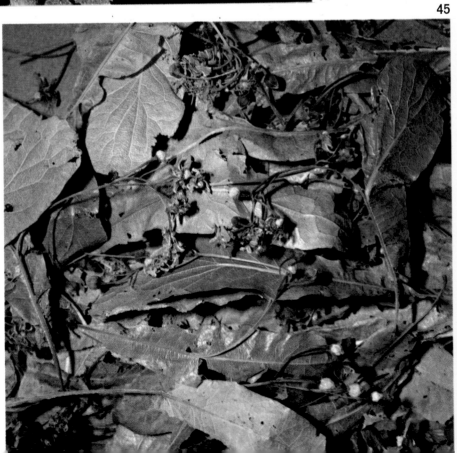

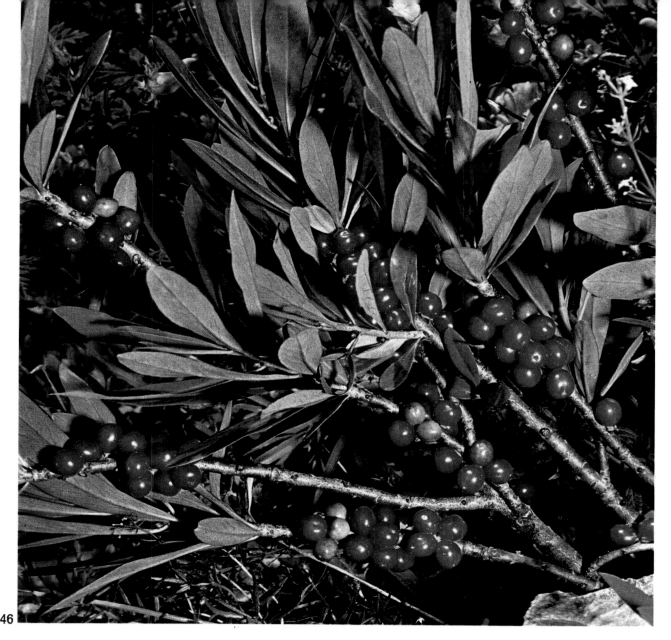

46

47

46 The mezereon (*Daphne mezereum*), otherwise called the spurge laurel, is cultivated for its beautiful flowers and berries – but these are extremely poisonous, as are all other parts of the plant. The fruit, a drupe, may be yellowish but is usually bright red. As a herbal, it can only be applied externally, in the form of a preparation made from the bark. This is a vesicant (blistering agent) and stimulant, used in liniments and for the treatment of certain types of ulcer.

47 Many species of the violet genus – this one is *Viola calcarata* – have similar herbal properties. For example, a decoction of the whole plant is used in the treatment of bronchitis, and contains an alkaloid used as purgative and emetic.

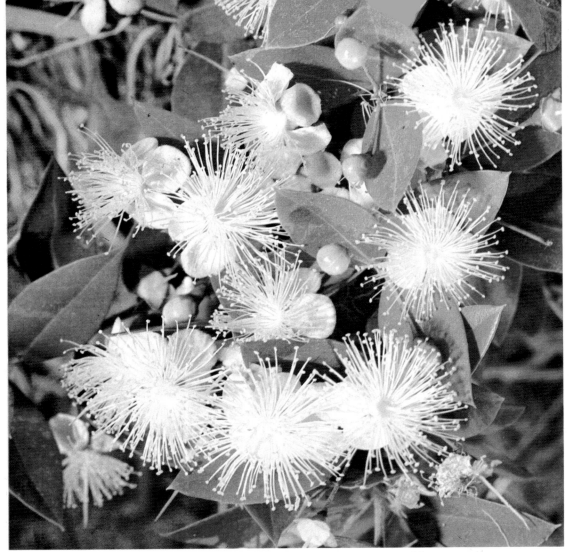

48

49

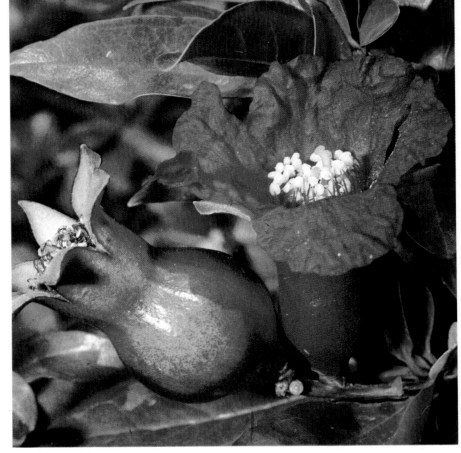

48 The myrtle (*Myrtus communis*) is an evergreen shrub, growing mainly in the Mediterranean region. Its pointed, scented leaves, white flowers and black berries make it an attractive plant, and it is the leaves that are used herbally. From them, both an infusion and a decoction can be obtained, for use as a gargle in stomatitis, or as a treatment for bronchitis and cystitis.

49 The pomegranate (*Punica granatum*) is a tree that grows to about fifteen feet. The fruits are well known and quite popular to eat; the flowers are red and attractive. An alkaloid, similar to hemlock, is obtained from the bark and used for the expulsion of tapeworms: a decoction is taken, and followed by a purgative, such as castor oil.

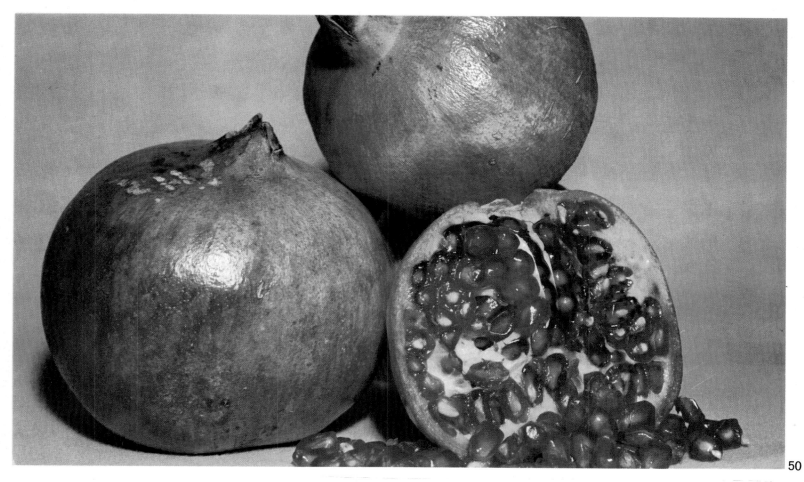

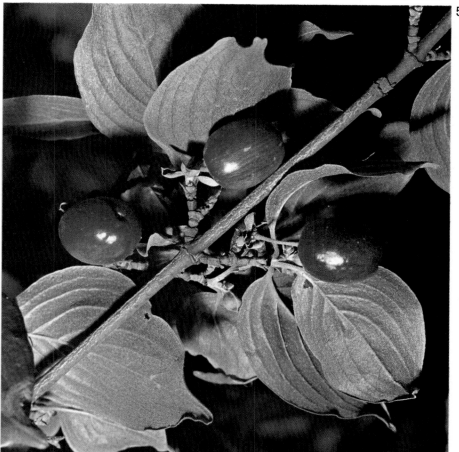

50 The fruit of the pomegranate, as well as its bark (see 49), has medicinal properties. A dried preparation of the rind has astringent properties, and is used to treat diarrhea and dysentery.

51 The cornelian cherry (*Cornus mas*) is a small tree, native to Europe and Asia, where it grows in woods and hedges or is cultivated as an ornamental plant. Its flowers are small and yellow, and the drupe fruits are red. They are edible, and may also be preserved for use as a mild astringent.

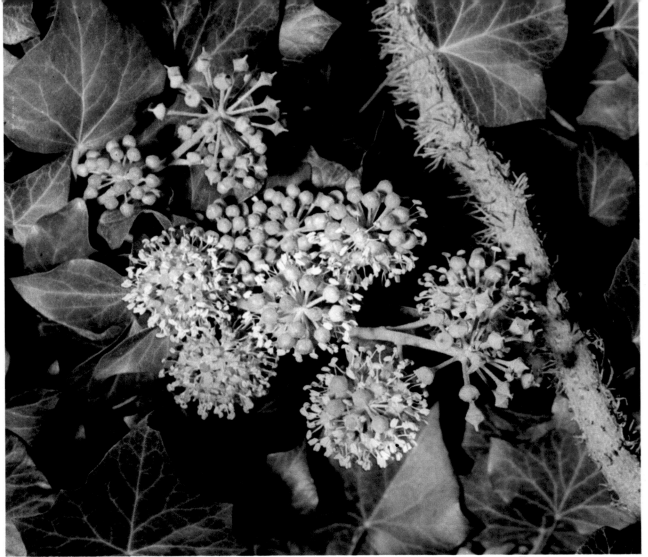

52

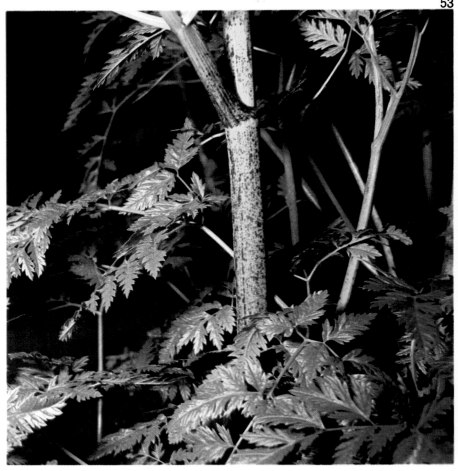

53

52 All the parts of the ivy (*Hedera helix*), especially the fruits, are poisonous. In herbal medicine, however, a small quantity of shedded leaves is immersed in hot water, to give an infusion which, despite being irritant and purgative, is believed to counteract catarrh, rheumatism and gout. Externally, the leaves may be incorporated into a poultice for use on ulcers and slow-healing wounds.

53 The hemlock (*Conium maculatum*) grows in shady, damp places; it has a hollow stem, finely divided leaves and small white flowers arranged in compound umbels. All parts of the plant contain an extremely poisonous alkaloid – the one that killed Socrates – but the fruit is the most potent source. Extracts containing the alkaloid may be used, with extreme care and under skilled supervision, for the alleviation of spasms in diseases such as chorea or parkinsonism, and as a sedative and analgesic. Extracts of the leaves are used externally in poultices, or in an ointment that relieves the discomfort of piles and pruritus ani.

54 *Heracleum sphondyllium* is variously known as the keck, hogweed, or cow parsley. Common by roadsides and in fields, it is a large umbelliferous plant, native to Europe and Africa, and introduced into North America. Both the fruit and the green parts are used, pulverized or in a decoction, for their sedative effect. It is related to the giant hogweed, reported to be a dangerous plant.

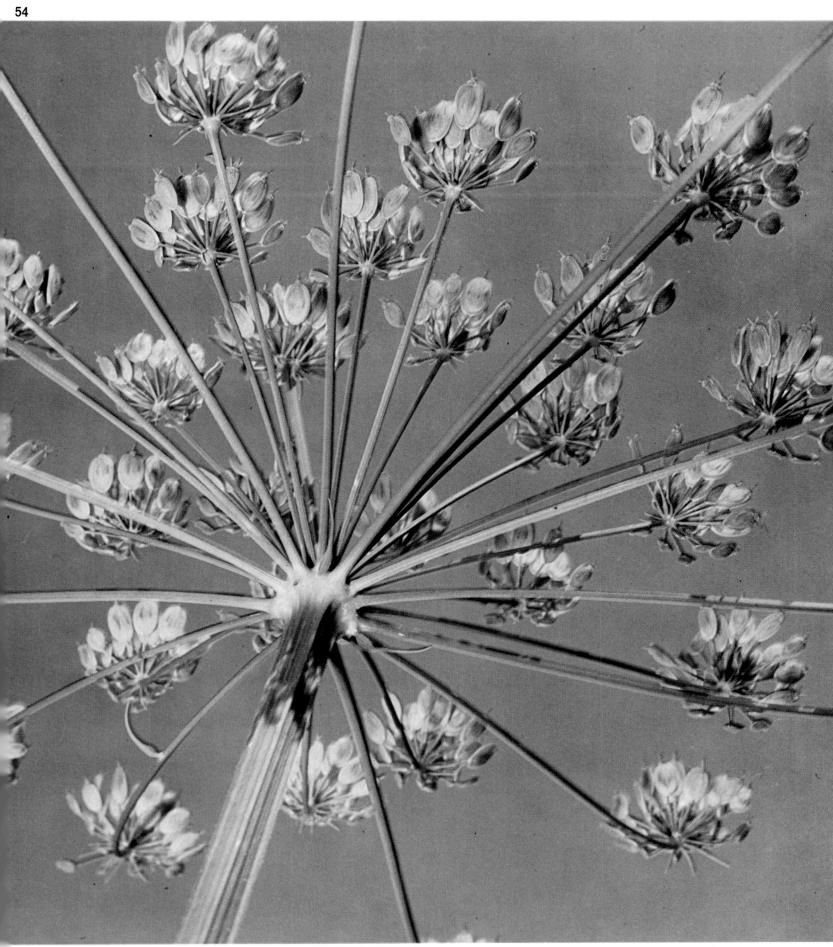

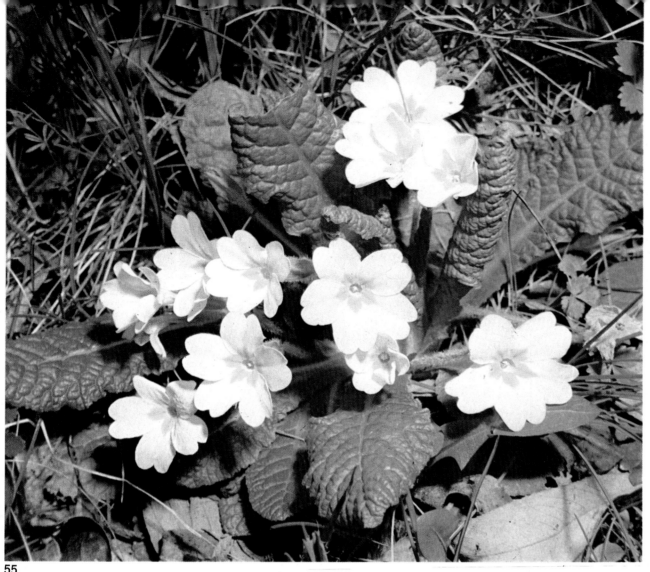

55

56

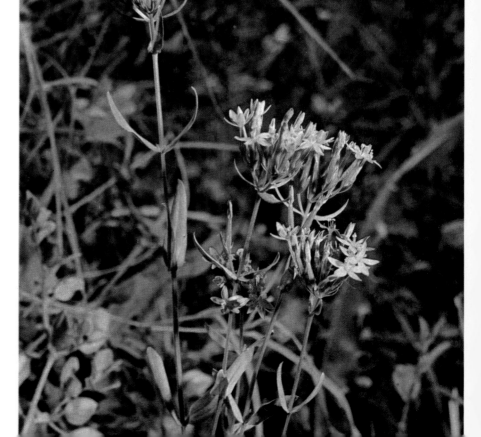

55 The primrose (*Primula vulgaris*), with its sulphur-yellow flowers, is a common sight in spring in many parts of Europe. Like many related species, it contains a saponin which has a diuretic and expectorant action, and has been made into a decoction for use in bronchitis. This preparation is made from the dried root and rhizome, and is generally similar to senega.

56 The medicinal properties of the centaury (*Centaurium erythraea*) have been known since classical times, and highly valued: hence its name, which means 'a hundred gold pieces'. It flowers in the summer, and it is this inflorescence that provides the active, bitter drug. As an infusion in wine, it has tonic and fever-reducing properties.

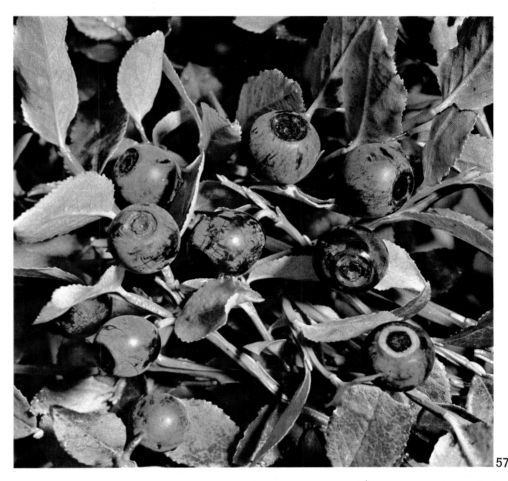

57

57 The genus *Vaccinium* consists of 300 to 400 species of evergreen or deciduous trees or shrubs, and includes the whortleberry, cranberry, blueberry and huckleberry. The species illustrated is *V. myrtillus*, the bilberry. Very many species, including this one, are cultivated for their edible fruit, which in this case is a blue colour, but may be red, purple or black. The fruits are generally rather acid, and can be used to make a preserve or a decoction with anti-diarrhea properties.

58 Another berry is the cowberry, or mountain cranberry (*Vaccinium vitisidaea*), which grows throughout Europe and the eastern states of America. The red, edible berries are rich in vitamins, and a decoction of the leaves forms a domestic remedy for diarrhea. This astringent preparation is also used against rheumatic conditions and gastrointestinal chills.

58

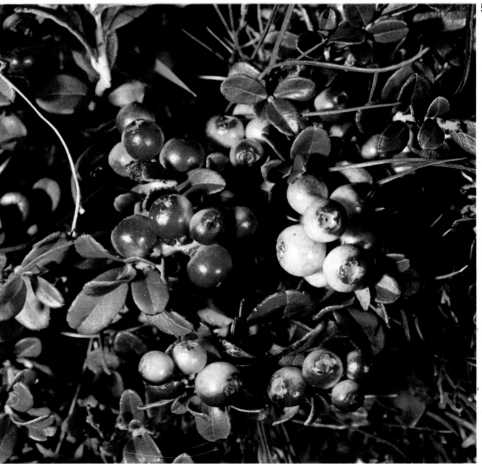

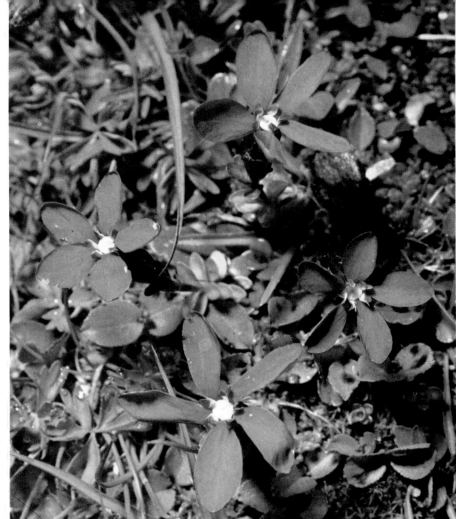

60

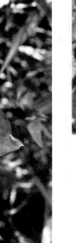

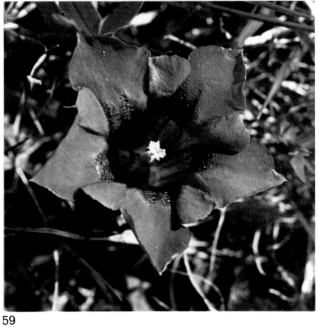

59

61

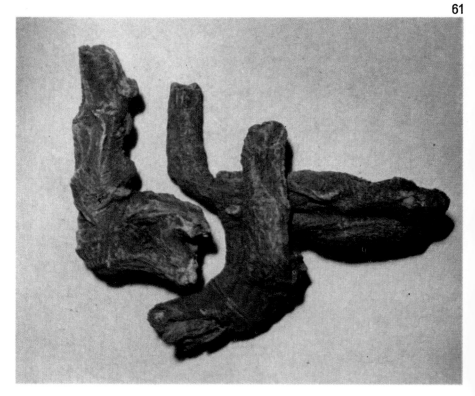

59–60–61 These are just three of the many species of *Gentiana* which have active herbal properties. They are the flowers of *G. acaulis* and *G. verna*, and the roots of *G. lutea*. In all cases, it is the root and the leaves which carry the therapeutic agent, a bitter glucoside with tonic and eupeptic properties. Many preparations are available, most of them made from *G. lutea*, which is the best source. (The well-known 'gentian violet' is not derived from this genus, despite its name.)

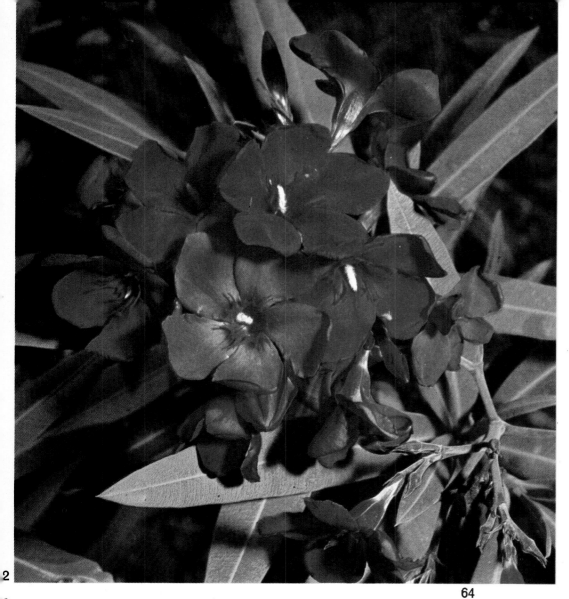

2

62–63–64 Three different varieties of the oleander (*Nerium oleander*); the white flower is much rarer than the pink ones. It is an evergreen shrub, native to southern Europe and North Africa, and often cultivated as an ornamental. The leaves, flowers and fruit are all potential sources of a mixture of four glycosides – collectively called oleandrin – whose effect is similar to that of strophanthin. It acts on the heart, in the manner of digitalis, strengthening a weak beat, but is more rapidly absorbed than digitalis and less cumulative. It is of some value, therefore, in medicine; as a herbal, it must be regarded with caution, as it can be very poisonous.

64

3

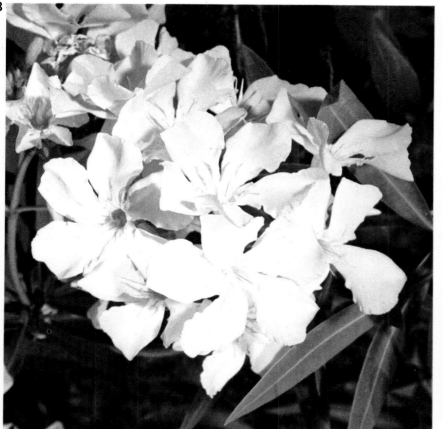

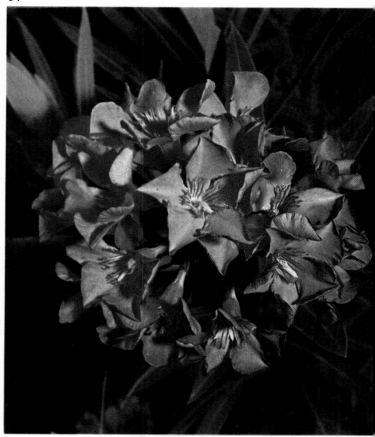

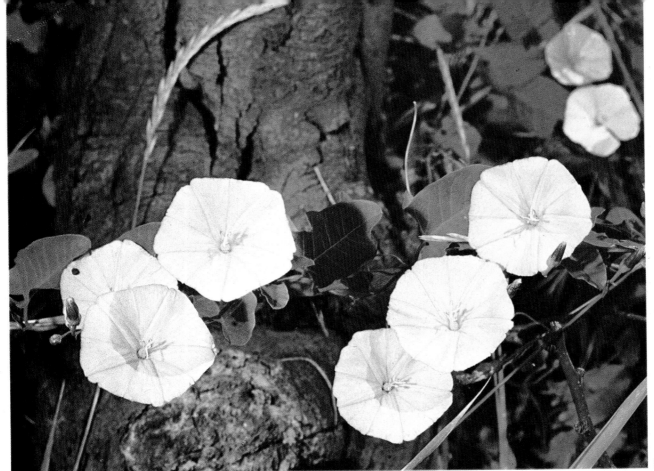

65

66

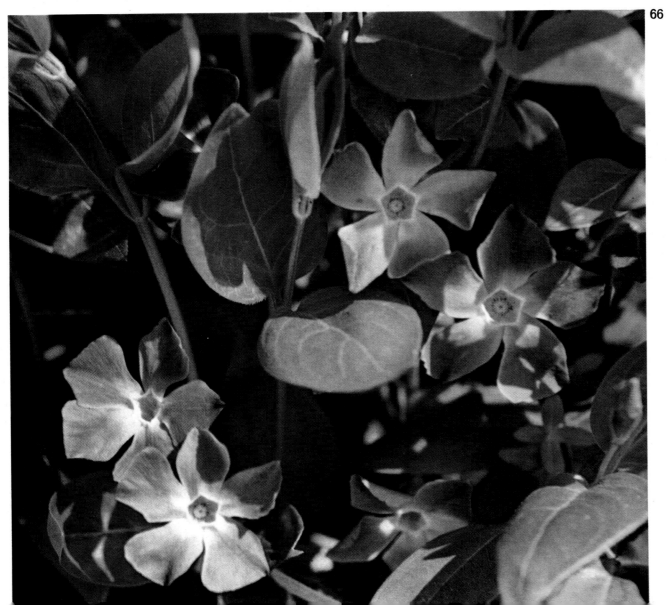

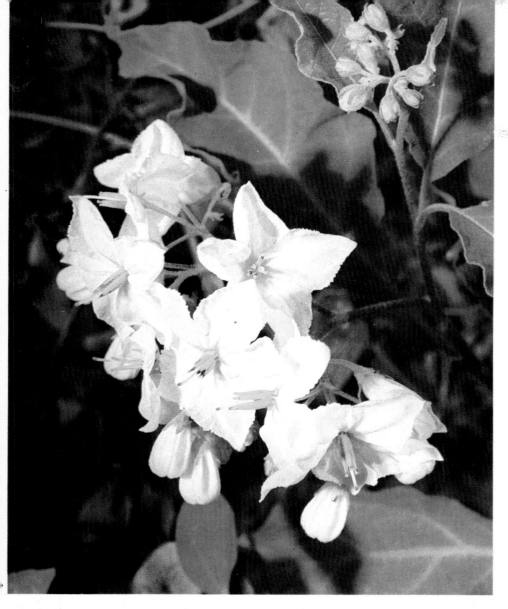

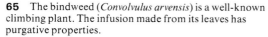

65 The bindweed (*Convolvulus arvensis*) is a well-known climbing plant. The infusion made from its leaves has purgative properties.

66 The genus *Vinca*, or periwinkle, is of considerable pharmacological interest. Two of its species, *V. minor* and *V. major*, both of them evergreen creepers, can provide a herbal that is used as a tonic and to counteract intestinal troubles. A third species, *V. rosea*, is a source of alkaloids used in the treatment of leukemia. The species illustrated is *V. major*.

67–68 Two typical examples of the flowering heads of plants of the Solanaceae family. This is the potato family, species of which are found in nearly every country of the world, and which originated in South America. Some species are agriculturally important: for example the potato (*Solanum tuberosum*), the tomato (*Lycopersicon esculentum*), and the aubergine (*Solanum melangena*). Others have a pharmaceutical value: the deadly nightshade (*Atropa bella-donna*), the henbane (*Hyoscyamus niger*), and the thornapple (*Datura stramonium*). (These are illustrated on the next page.) Even the edible types of Solanaceae can be poisonous, since the green parts of their tubers contain solanin, a toxic alkaloid. This applies to potatoes, of which the green parts should always be discarded.

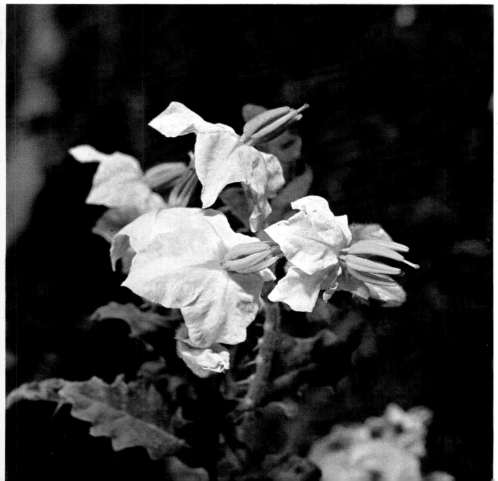

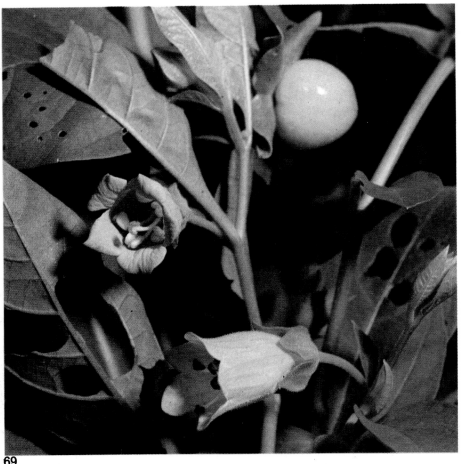

69

70

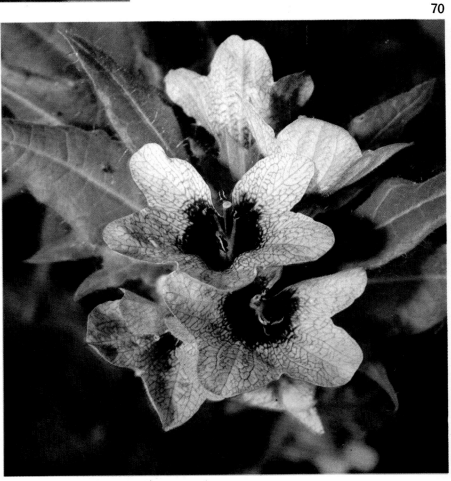

69 The deadly nightshade, or belladonna (*Atropa bella-donna*) derives its poetic name from the fact that ladies once used to put drops of the extract in their eyes to make them wide and beautiful (hence *bella donna*: beautiful lady). This occurred because of the action of the drug (known as belladonna in its crude form, and atropine when purified), which is present in the leaves, roots and seeds, and which acts on nerve endings to interrupt their normal functions. Medicinally it is a useful drug, but it is extremely powerful, and all but the expert pharmacist should regard belladonna as a deadly poison.

70 The henbane (*Hyoscyamus niger*) has a yellowish flower with a purple centre, and soft, hairy leaves. The drug obtained from its seeds is an alkaloid similar to those present in belladonna, but with an even stronger narcotic effect. Like belladonna, it is useful in medicine.

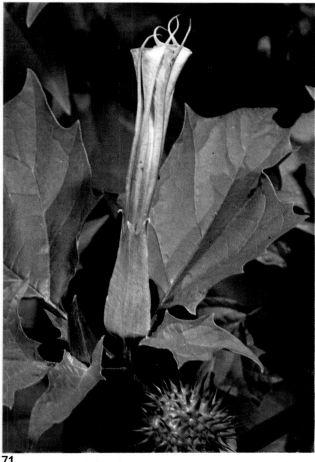

71

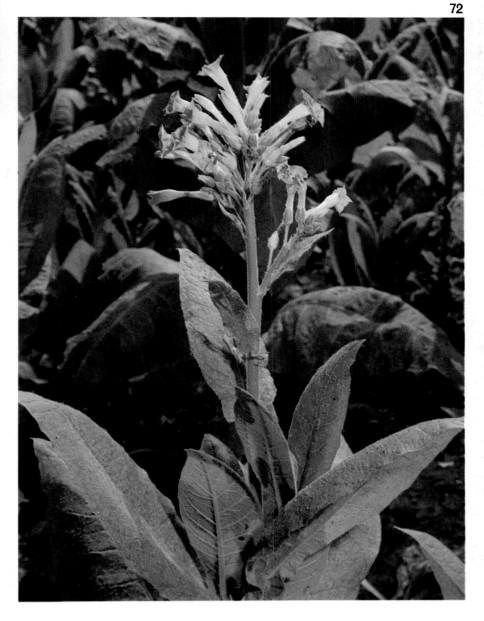

72

71 The thornapple (*Datura stramonium*) is a source of yet another mixture of alkaloids, chiefly atropine and hyoscyamine, giving it similar properties to those of belladonna and henbane. The uses of the drug are similar too: for gastric ulcers, parkinsonism, etc. It has also been incorporated in cigarettes for asthmatics, but it is believed that the effect of the smoke makes this measure counter-productive, particularly when bronchitis is present.

72 The famous, or infamous, tobacco plant, *Nicotiana tabacum*. It contains nicotine, an alkaloid which is so toxic that preparations of the plant are nowadays used only as parasiticides in veterinary medicine and agriculture. The only other pharmacological interest in the plant is the fact that so many people smoke dried preparations of its leaves: the nicotine obtained in this way has a short-term effect, and possibly long-term influences also. The irritation of the smoke and some of its constituents cause cancer, and have been implicated in other diseases.

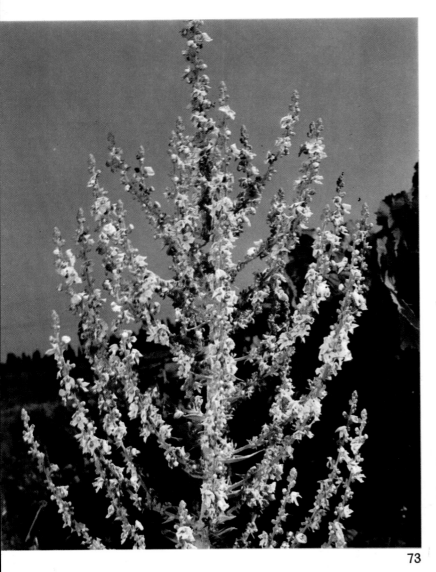

73

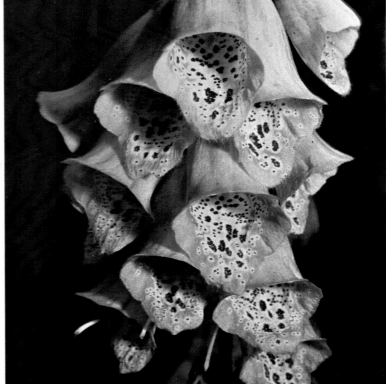

74

73 The leaves and flowers of *Verbascum phlomoides* can be made into a soothing decoction. The plant grows in dry, stony, uncultivated areas, and its use in bronchitis has been widespread in the countries of Europe. For this and other throat, bronchial or pulmonary complaints, its value is solely that of a demulcent.

74 Perhaps the most famous of all medicinal plants is the purple foxglove, *Digitalis purpurea*. The typical arrangement of the pendulous flowers makes this and other foxgloves both attractive and easily recognizable; the purple foxglove is particularly striking. The drug is obtained from the leaves, and is a mixture of glycosides, together called digitalis, which has a powerful action on the heart. In heart failure it is often the best, or the only, life-saving drug. Its primary action is to increase the force of the heart beat: this, in turn, increases the amount of blood that the heart is pumping, slows the heart rate, decreases the enlargement of the heart, and helps the body to dispose of excess fluid through the kidneys. Used over a long time, digitalis can have toxic effects; but for the acute case of heart failure, it is without equal.

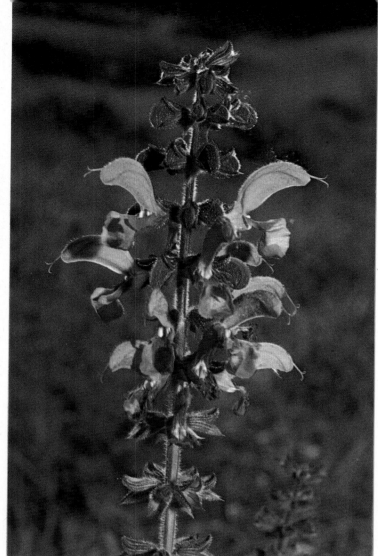

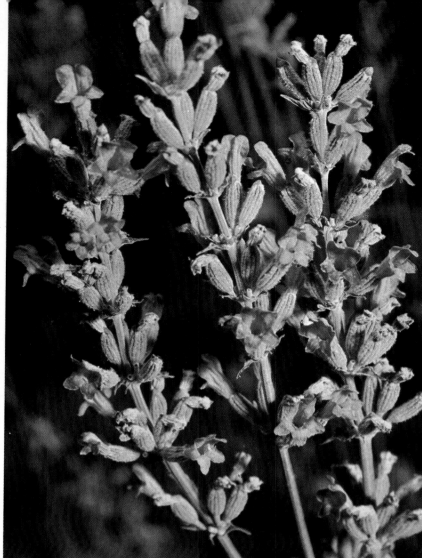

75 76

77

75 Rather a long step down from digitalis, in the herbalist's and the pharmacist's list, is the meadow glory plant (*Salvia pretensis*). In parts of Europe and North Africa, where it is a native species, it is claimed to have stomachic properties, but these are unsubstantiated. A related species, *S. sclarea*, is also thought to promote the activity of the stomach, and in this case the plant is also cultivated for its pleasant smell.

76 The lavender plant (*Lavandula spica* and *L. latifolia*) is best known for its extremely attractive smell; indeed, this property is made use of in many preparations of herbals and cosmetics. In addition, an infusion made from the flowers is an effective antispasmodic, and other preparations have been used in herbal remedies for migraine and baldness. Lavender oil, distilled from the flowers, is a carminative.

77 The shrub rosemary (*Rosmarinus officinalis*) has several uses, and is often cultivated. The pleasantly smelling leaves, useful to the cook, are herbals to induce sweating or menstruation; and the oil extracted from the flowering tops is used as a carminative and in hair lotions.

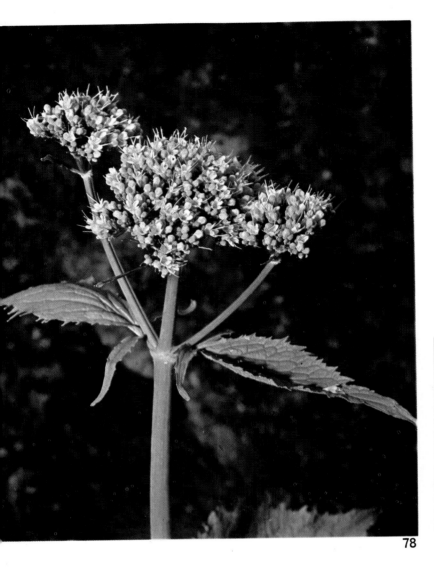

78

78 The pharmacological activity of the valerian (*Valeriana officinalis*) is much greater in the fresh plant than in the dried one. The active principle is contained in the rhizome, and its sedative and antispasmodic effect is used in treating hysteria. It also acts as a carminative, and can be obtained as an infusion, a macerate, or a powder. There are almost two hundred species of valerian, all with more or less the same herbal properties.

79 The most striking feature of the teasel (*Dipsacus fullonum*) is its ovoid flower head, with the stiff spines. These are still used today in the wool industry, for raising the nap of cloth. Its pharmacological activity, as a stomachic, is contained in the roots.

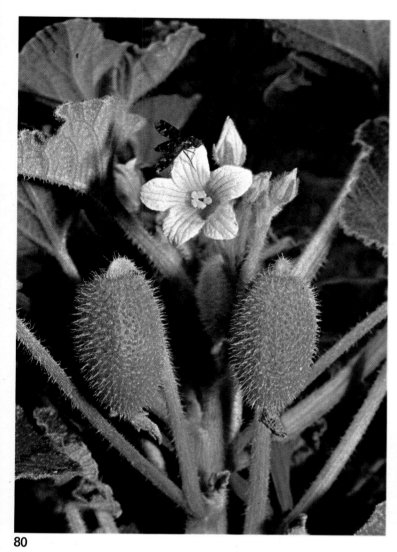

80

81

80 *Ecballium elaterium* is called the squirting cucumber because of the way it disperses its seeds: when the fruit is mature, it detaches itself from the stalk in an explosive manner, scattering the seeds over some distance. To obtain an active extract of the plant, however, the immature fruit must be taken; a cut in this releases a fluid which congeals to form a substance called elaterium. It is a strong and rather unpredictable purgative, certainly effective but quite liable to cause prostration if taken too often or in excessive amounts.

81 The bark of *Cinchona* is important as a source of the drug quinine, which was for many years the only effective means of combating malaria, and which is still used for this purpose today. The alkaloid is extracted from the bark, along with others which can play a part in controlling heart palpitations.

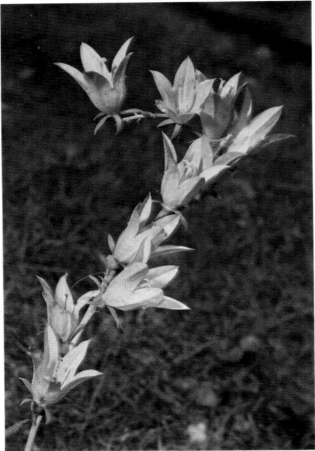

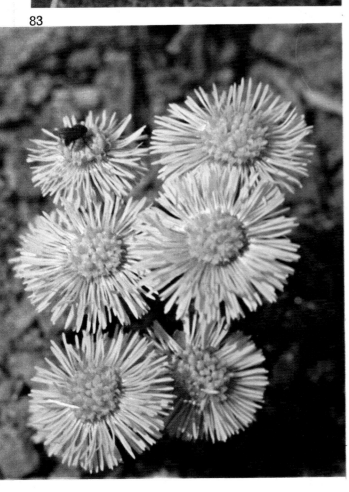

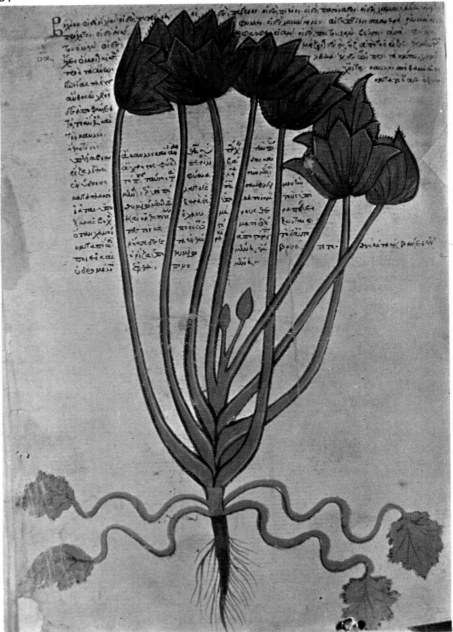

82 This pretty blue plant of the hedgerows is the rampion (*Campanula rapunculus*). Its fleshy roots are rich in a starch-like substance called inulin – the same carbohydrate as in Jerusalem artichokes – and the aerial parts of the plant can be made into an infusion and used as a mouthwash.

83 The coltsfoot (*Tussilago farfara*) is another common wild flower in Europe, and in North America, to which it has been introduced. It flowers in spring, and both the inflorescence and the leaves, which appear later, can be used to prepare a cough mixture with expectorant and soothing properties.

84 The same plant, the coltsfoot, was depicted by Dioscorides in the fourteenth century, along with an account of its curative and mythical properties.

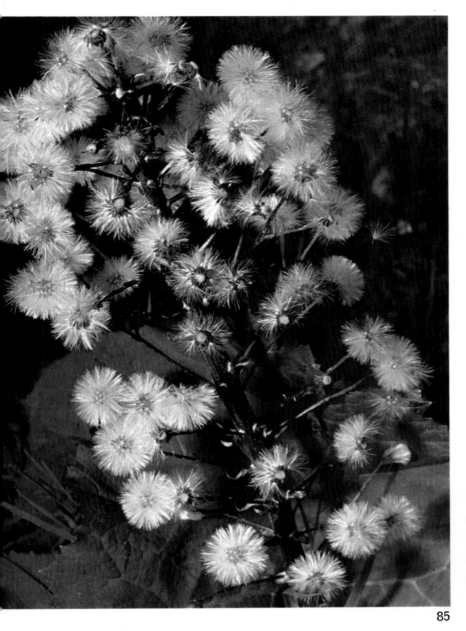

85

85 The delicate, windblown butterbur (*Patasites hybridus*) grows in wet places, particularly the banks of streams. The leaves and the rhizomes are collected and used on skin wounds and abscesses, while the roots and the rhizomes – if collected in early spring – are said to be stomachic and anti-arthritic in action.

86 The arnica, or mountain tobacco (*Arnica montana*) is a European plant that grows on mountains. A drug prepared from the flowers and rhizomes is used externally on bruises and other skin ailments, but is only safe when the skin is unbroken, since the tincture is rather poisonous. For the same reason, internal use of arnica herbals is possible only when they are very weak; such solutions are thought to have a tonic and stimulating effect, and have been used in cases of bronchial asthma.

86

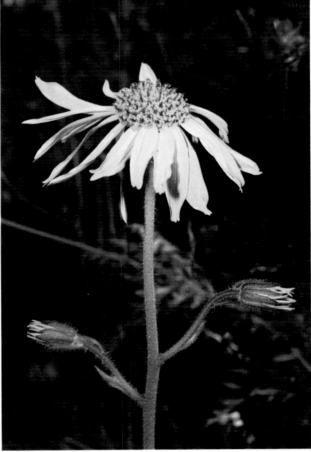

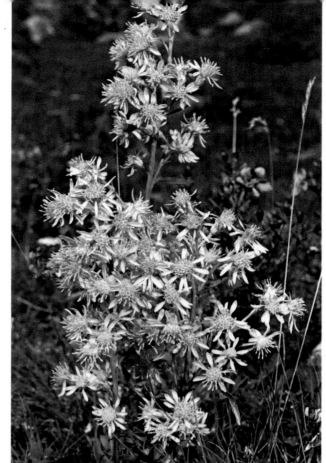

87 The golden rod (*Solidago virgaurea*) grows in North America, Asia and Europe, usually on banks, cliffs, dunes and mountains. It is also cultivated as a garden plant. One part used in herbal medicine is the flower, from which an infusion can be made. This acts as a diuretic. On the other hand, the whole plant may be prepared into a mouthwash to soothe a sore throat or mouth.

88 This plant of the *Chrysanthemum* genus is the tansy (*C. vulgare*). It is very poisonous, but may be used – with great care – to rid the body of worms. In this respect, it is effective against nematode worms and pinworms; for the latter, it is used in the form of an enema.

87

88

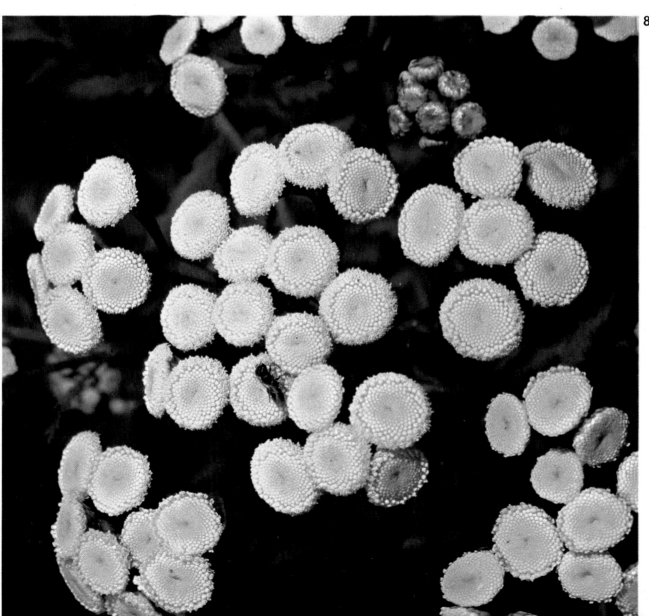

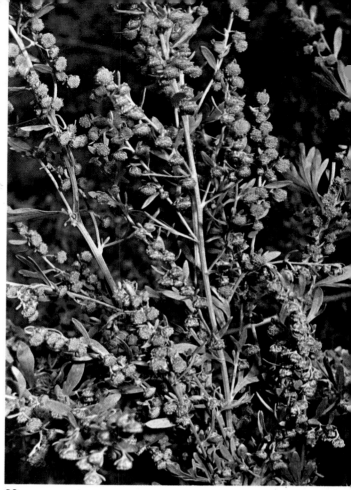

89 The wormwood (*Artemisia absinthium*) has caused a great deal of trouble. It is widespread in Europe; a related plant, the sage brush, being more common in North America. The flowers and leaves of the wormwood can be used to prepare a stimulant, bitter herbal preparation, which has been used as a tonic and stimulant for many hundreds of years. It was the main ingredient in the drink absinthe, which was responsible for a great deal of misery and controversy, particularly during the nineteenth century, until it was eventually declared illegal. The problem is that the drug is addictive, and if it is taken regularly it causes poisoning of the central nervous system, typified by convulsions.

90 The long history of the use of *Artemisia absinthium* is exemplified by this drawing of the plant, again from the fourteenth-century work of Dioscorides. The notes describe its properties, including an apparently effective cure for the bites of rats and spiders.

89

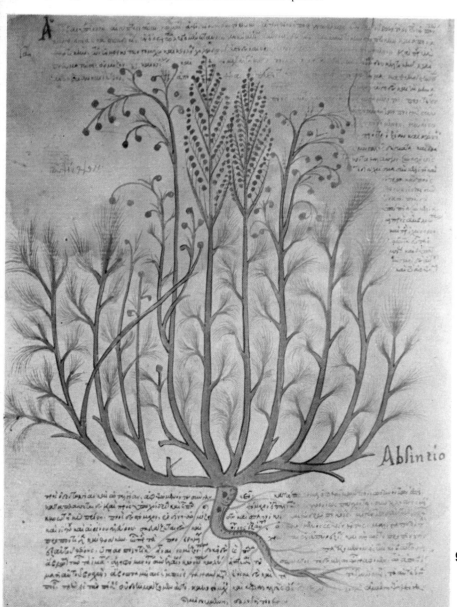

90

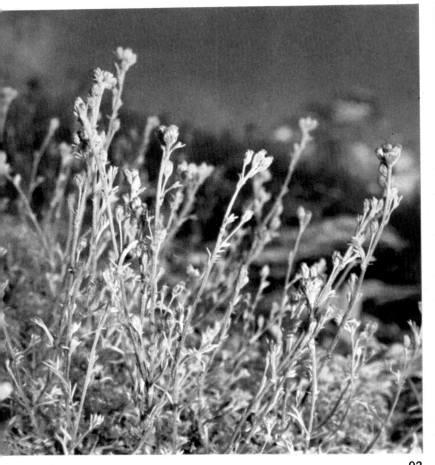

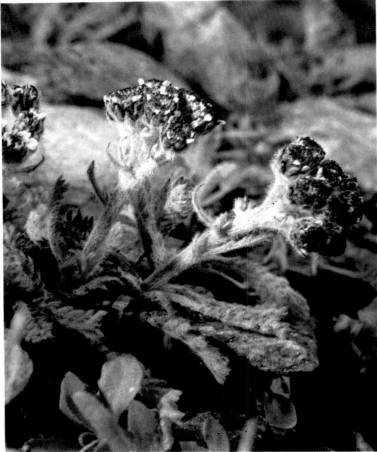

93

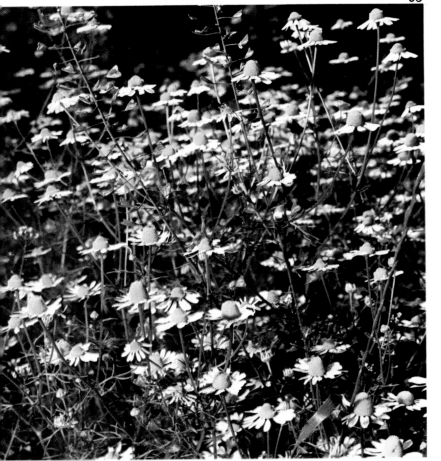

91   Another species of *Artemisia* is *A. mutellina*. Along with the two hundred or so other species of this genus, it has some properties in common with the notorious wormwood, and may still be used in certain areas of the wine and spirits business.

92   This mountain plant is *Achillea nana*, one of the many species of *Achillea* to have been used medicinally. Others, like *A. moschata*, *A. atrata*, etc, share its bitter alkaloids and its stomachic properties, and are used in the manufacture of liqueurs. *A. millefolium* is the source of an infusion with diaphoretic, stimulant and hemostatic properties.

93   The wild chamomile (*M. recutita*) is similar to *Anthemis nobilis*, the well-known plant from which chamomile tea and other preparations are obtained. *Matricaria* is often found growing wild, although it is sometimes cultivated, and has found use as an anti-neuralgic, an anti-asthmatic, and in the treatment of gastrointestinal spasm. These effects are achieved by an infusion of the flowers.

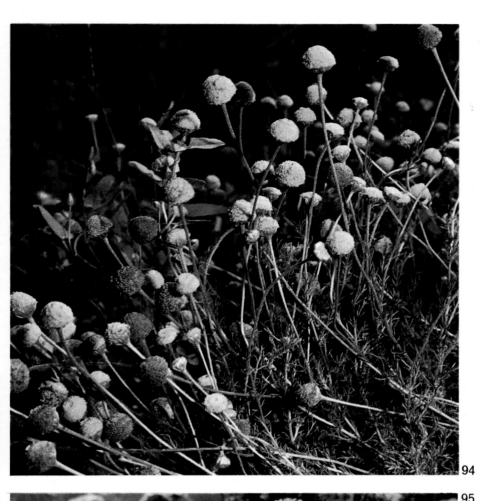

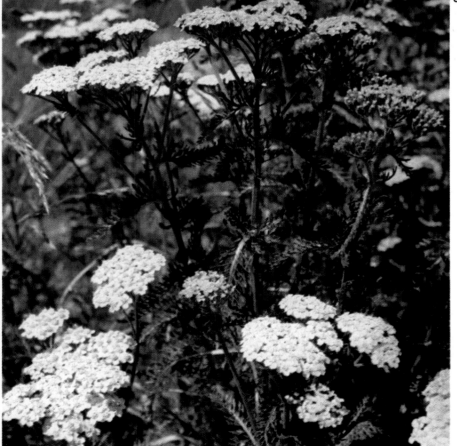

94 This is another species of *Matricaria*, with similar properties to the wild chamomile. It is the pineapple weed (*M. matricaroides*), whose heads, unlike those of *M. recutita* and *Anthemis nobilis*, have no ray florets.

95 This is the yarrow, or milfoil (*Achillea millefolium*), referred to earlier (see 92). The aerial parts of the plants are used herbally to provide an infusion with properties similar to those of chamomile: it is diaphoretic, hemostatic, stimulant and stomachic. Many herbal remedies incorporate the yarrow.

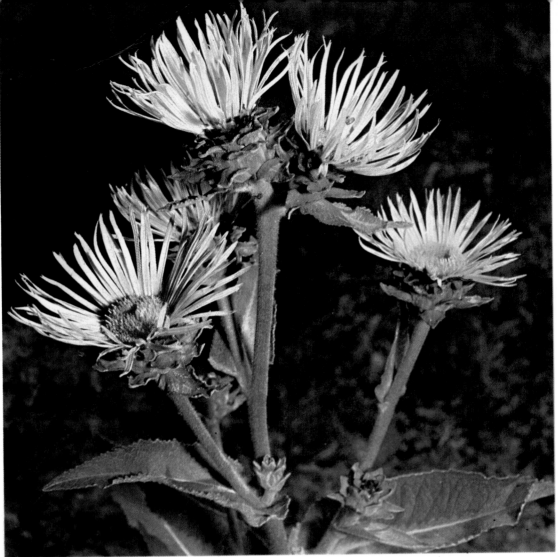

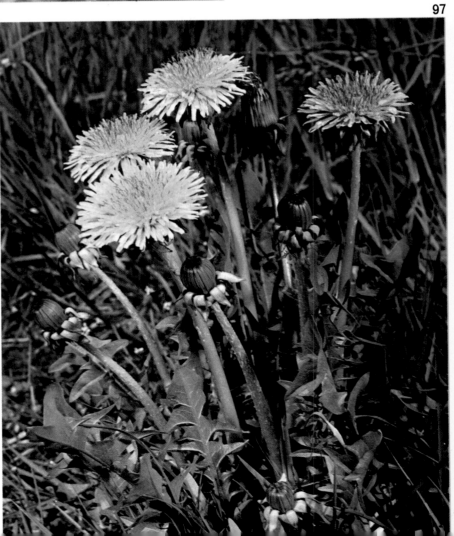

96 The elecampene (*Inula helenium*), like the rampion (see 82), is a source of the carbohydrate inulin. This may be eaten, but is more commonly used as an expectorant or externally as an anti-irritant. In hospital work, inulin is used in an important test of the function of the kidneys.

97 One of the most common and best known of all wild flowers is the dandelion (*Taracaxum officinale*). Its leaves may be eaten, and its roots have been used in all kinds of herbal remedies for very many years. The main properties of the root, which may be taken as an extract, a juice, or in dandelion coffee, are those of a mild laxative, diuretic and stomachic.

98 Apart from its glorious, tall beauty, the most important thing about the sunflower (*Helianthus annuus*) is its seeds. The oil extracted from them is of great commercial importance, for it is used as a cooking oil, in the preparation of soft (unsaturated) margarines, and in several other ways in the food industry. Medicinally, this oil is a valuable substitute for hard fats, and has also been used as a herbal to evacuate the gall bladder. In addition, an infusion of the outer flowers and the leaves of the sunflower is said to be effective against certain lung conditions.

99 The stemless thistle (*Carlina acaulis*) is not necessarily stemless, although it usually lives up to its name. In autumn, the root is very rich in active chemicals, and it is sometimes harvested at this time and prepared into a herbal tonic, diaphoretic and diuretic.

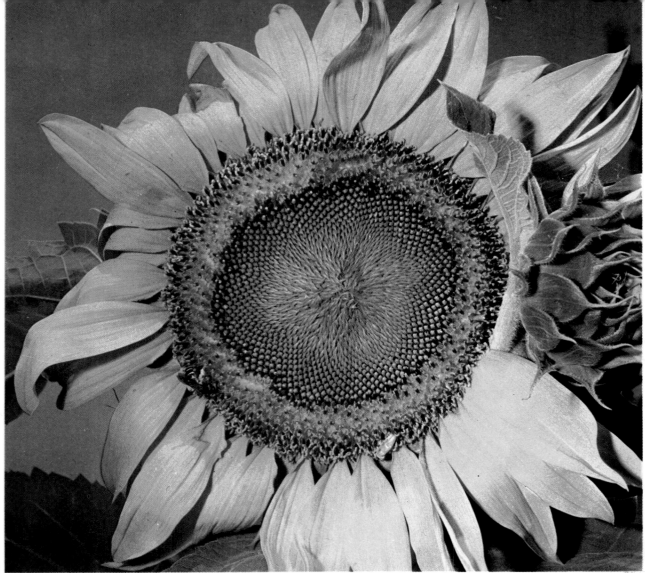
98

99
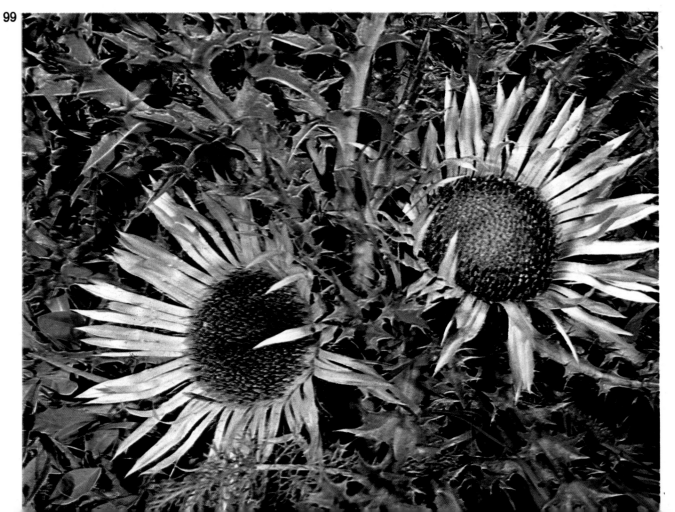

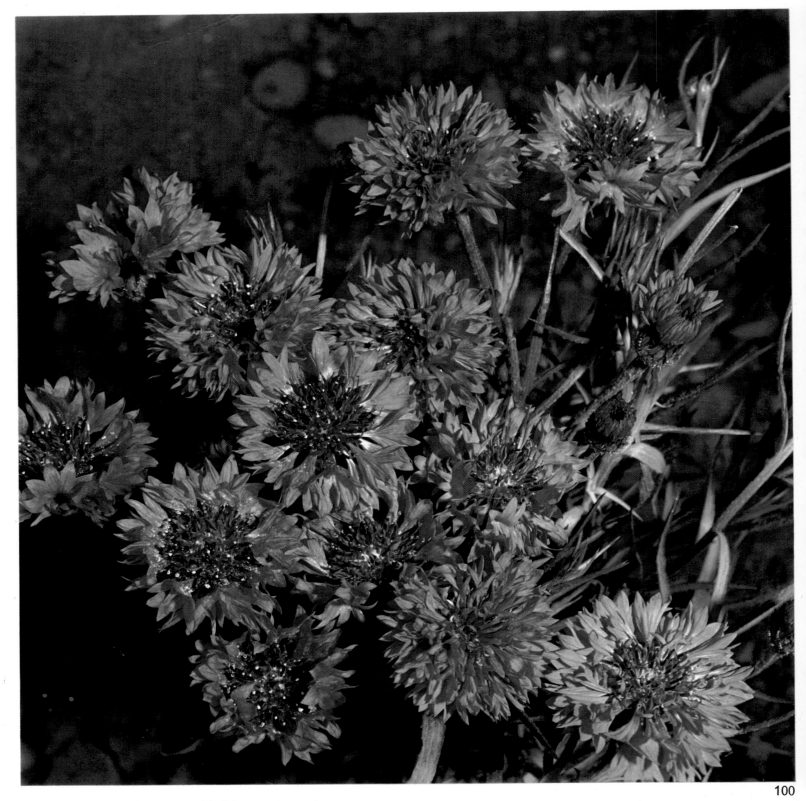

100 The cornflower (*Centauria cyanus*) is of the same genus as the centaury (see 56), but has not the same medicinal properties. Its main use is in the preparation of a decoction, which is used as an eyewash against conjunctivitis, while an infusion of the plant provides a cough mixture.

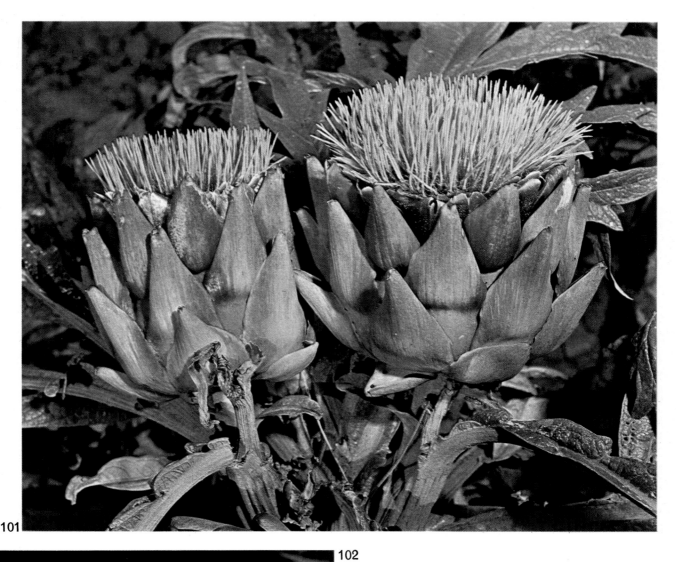

101

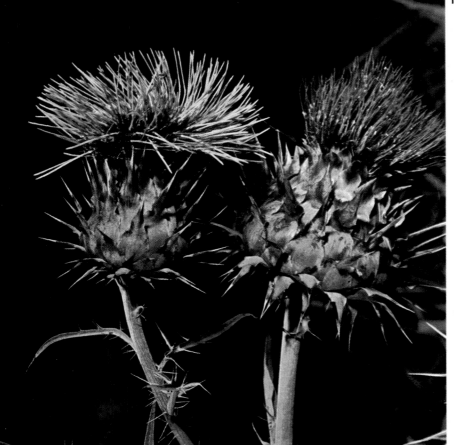

102

101 The globe artichoke (*Cynara cardunculus*, var *scolymus*) is well known for its delicate taste, and the roots and leaves have therapeutic properties, acting particularly on the liver.

102 Similar in its herbal properties is the wild variety of the artichoke (*Cynara cardunculus* var *altilis*). It differs in appearance from the cultivated form, especially in the spikiness of its flowering head.

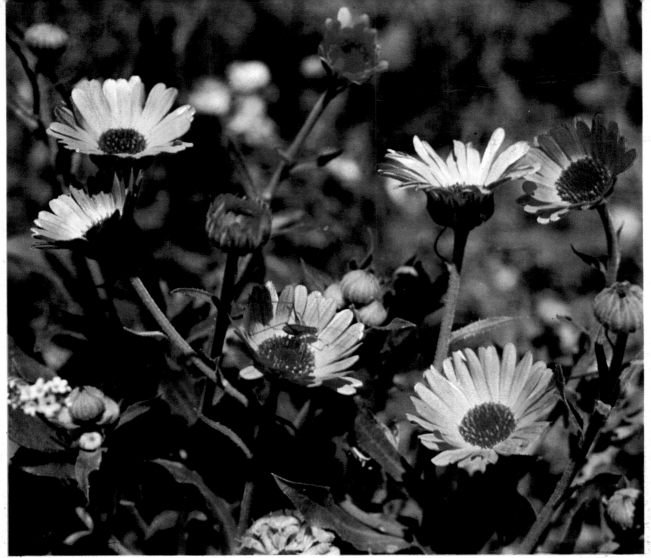

103

104

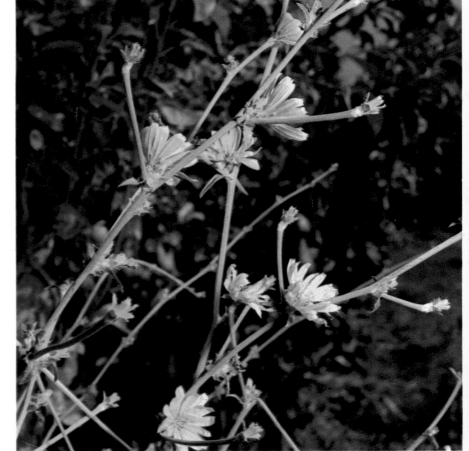

103 The large, yellow-orange flower heads of the marigold (*Calendula officinalis*) are rich in various pigments used in ointments for wounds, sores, chilblains and burns, while a fluid extract of the plant is said to stimulate the secretion of bile. The same bitter principle in the flowers has been claimed to exhibit diaphoretic, diuretic and stimulant properties, and an aqueous extract has been shown to have a slight activity against cancer.

104 *Cichorium intybus* is the chicory, whose essence is often used as an addition to coffee. An infusion or decoction of the root is said to stimulate appetite, and to alleviate constipation in children. The fresh roots are claimed to be depurative; while the leaves, eaten as a salad, can be used to counter high blood pressure, or as a poultice on skin ulcers.